A Trail of Envy

M.D. MacGregor, MD

Order this book online at www.trafford.com
or email orders@trafford.com

Most Trafford titles are also available at major online book retailers.

© Copyright 2010 M.D. MacGregor, MD.
All rights reserved. No part of this publication may be reproduced, stored in a retrieval system, or transmitted, in any form or by any means, electronic, mechanical, photocopying, recording, or otherwise, without the written prior permission of the author.

Printed in Victoria, BC, Canada.

ISBN: 978-1-4269-2971-7

Our mission is to efficiently provide the world's finest, most comprehensive book publishing service, enabling every author to experience success. To find out how to publish your book, your way, and have it available worldwide, visit us online at www.trafford.com

Trafford rev. 4/30/2010

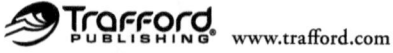 www.trafford.com

North America & international
toll-free: 1 888 232 4444 (USA & Canada)
phone: 250 383 6864 ♦ fax: 812 355 4082

Acknowledgements

I would never have been the free spirit capable of giving special care to my patients were it not for my mother and father. They were unselfish with their love and generous with their trust. I was allowed to be a free spirit from infancy. I respected and pondered written knowledge and formal training, but was never blindsided by it. My expertise expanded everyday. I learned as much from my patients as they learned from me. I lived by the dictum, *"First of all do no harm…"*

My six children deserve gratitude for trying to understand their unconventional father. I have always loved all of them unconditionally. Susan in particular, I wish to credit for unwittingly providing the prologue for this book by handing me a recent horoscope reading. She and I have become closer than ever this past year while she has been helping me adjust to solitary living. It was she who invented the quote, "The world according to Malcolm" and with pride repeats it often to bolster my spirit. Lisa Berger, a lovely girl and a laptop whiz connected me to the digital world and made this book printable.

Preface

I was privileged to have practiced medicine for 35 years during its golden age. Penicillin had recently been discovered and technology was adequate but not overwhelming. The legal profession was reluctant at that point in time to advertise for clients, practice cookbook medicine in the courtroom and lobby overtly in Washington, DC.

Medicare and government regulations were just beginning to find traction and interfere with patient care. All in all, I was free to render personal service that was more effective and economical. I look back with great satisfaction and am happy that the defensive, impersonal care of today was after my time.

This is the story of the private battle incessantly fought to fulfill my destiny.

Prologue

MY HOROSCOPE READING:

"You are one of a kind. You think you can't possibly be that unique, but you are. You're seeing the world differently than anyone else is seeing it. If someone says it can't be done, take that as your invitation to do it."

MY POEM:

Malcolm's World

Dare to set the bar at good
To see a world of possibility
Such honesty is seen as strange
Down a road of misunderstood

Oft times I do forget
To remind myself over again
Can I balance on this perch
An uncomfortable place to set

Inborn spirit controls the day
No choice is given me
Wrapped in my self-made cocoon
I dare the world to sway

Persistence is my sky
Steadfast forward all I know
Doubters lick their wounds
To wonder what passed by

A Trail of Envy

CHAPTER I

In the Beginning

Ray's powerful grip held the 1920 Dodge touring car on the windswept road that black November night. He hunched forward over the wooden steering wheel, straining to see through the sheet of rain that the struggling wipers could not carry from the windshield.

Ray was the youngest of Emma's eleven siblings. When their mother died prematurely, Emma, the oldest daughter, took her place as the stay at home caretaker. She raised Ray, who was only four years old when their mother died. He would always look upon Emma as his mother and worship her. He was now twenty-eight and fresh out of the Navy with a lithe muscular body and tattooed arms. Ray had been the Pacific Coast Light-Weight Boxing Champion while in the service. His good looks and carefree nature endeared him to the young women who crossed his path. In fact, he was likeable and interesting to everyone.

Scottie, in the front passenger seat, stiffened his legs against the floorboards. He had always been afraid in a car and would never take the wheel himself. An accident many years ago when he had been driving sealed his fate. Emma always drove their car when she and Scottie were alone. His demonstrative fear tested their marriage continually.

Scottie had met Emma's father, Albert when they worked together on the railroad in Centralia, Washington. Albert invited Scottie to dinner one night where he enjoyed Emma's cooking and company. Albert felt sorry for Scottie, who had, in his estimation, been batching it far too long. Scottie's wife had walked out two years earlier, leaving him to raise their twelve-year-old daughter, Kathryn. That dinner led to Scottie and Emma's marriage in 1922. Emma took on the monumental task of mothering the teen-aged Kathryn. Her patience was sorely tested but her kind heart and gentle nature tamed Kathryn's wildness. Emma and Scottie's son, Malcolm, was born on December 9, 1925.

In the backseat, Emma and Aunt Ted, Scottie's older sister, were blissfully unaware of any danger since they could not see what lay ahead. Emma cradled Malcolm, then eleven months old, in her lap. She held him proudly and securely. He was her first born, a healthy lovable baby with a quick smile. She adored him. Emma, who at the tender age of fourteen, had traded sisterhood for motherhood because of her devotion to her brother Ray. Malcolm was the beneficiary of that premature experience and her well directed love shaped his early years.

"Scottie! Stop pushing on those floorboards for God's sake," Ray shouted, his voice filled with frustration. "You're making me crazy!"

"Then slow down, I can't see a thing out there," Scottie yelled back at him, bracing himself even more securely with his hands against the dash as icy fingers of panic raced through him.

"For Christ's sake, you're not driving, I am," Ray shot back. "Close your eyes and pray if you want to help." Trying to regain his composure, he added, "Just try to relax Scottie, I am only going 20 miles an hour." Ray adjusted and tightened his grip to reassure his nervous passenger, but deep inside waves of apprehension coursed through him too.

"Calm down Ray and pay attention to the road," Aunt Ted offered helpfully from behind him. Ray was sweating now because he could only see the dark road when the weak headlights caught an occasional reflection from the blurred yellow centerline. There were no white edge markers to direct him.

He was not aware that the road curved slightly on its approach to the Toutle River bridge dead ahead. He corrected too late. The fragile bumper of the Dodge was no match for its heavy 12 x 12 timber construction. With the sickening crunch of buckling metal, the car stopped instantly, propelling those inside against the flimsy side curtains abruptly tearing them from the car. Scottie, still gripping the dash, stayed in next to a stunned and momentarily speechless Ray, who had braced himself with the steering wheel. Aunt Ted was catapulted out onto the rough unforgiving pavement. Emma, buffered by Ted ended up on the floor behind the front seat. She righted herself, screaming hysterically, "Where's Malcolm? Where's my baby?"

Scottie leaped out into the blackness, stumbling over Ted, who was staggering to her feet. He reached out to steady her. "Did you see the baby?" he pleaded hopefully. Rain and blood ran in intermingling rivulets down her bewildered face. Scottie shook her, "Did you see the baby?"

"I think Malcolm flew out behind me," she stammered haltingly as she sagged to the pavement, holding her head.

Scottie dropped to his knees, groping the pavement in ever widening circles, while Emma's screams continued to punctuate the growing pandemonium.

"Are you hurt Emma?" Ray asked, torn between attending her and joining in the search.

She managed a "No, I'm alright…" as sobs wracked her thin body and she began to shake. "Don't worry about me…just find Malcolm… please."

Ray joined the distraught Scottie in the search. "He's not here! He's gone!" Scottie cried helplessly.

Ray stopped and listened for the cries of the baby, but heard only the rain-swollen river, now barely a few feet below the bridge. There was no sound except the river's thunderous roar. A sickening thought overwhelmed Ray; if Malcolm had flown more than thirty feet, he was in that churning river now, carried downstream and gone forever. He kept these grim thoughts to himself as he felt his way to the bridge. Not knowing what else to do, he explored the overlooked two foot plank projection beyond the bridge supports. He was stunned, when after what seemed like forever, his searching fingers felt a squirming bundle. A cry of relief escaped his lips as he felt the buttons of Malcolm's sweater. It had hooked on a spike projecting ominously through the plank and he lay secured as safely as if he were still cradled in his mother's arms. Carefully, he lifted the baby free.

Ray was crying now as he carried Malcolm to Emma. Trembling, he handed his precious package into her waiting arms. "Here is your baby, Emma…he's okay…not a scratch."

Pure joy replaced the tragedy that had been etched on Scottie's face only moments before. He grasped Ray's shoulder, "How can I ever thank you Ray? There are no words that can say what I'm feeling right now…I can only say thank you." Bowing his head, he whispered, "and thank you, God." Ray and Scottie held on to one another to keep from collapsing with relief.

"We need help for Ted now," Scottie said, regaining his composure, "She's hurt bad."

Aunt Ted was slumped over; sitting with her head between her badly scraped and bloodied knees. Ray assured her that Malcolm was okay and he proceeded to wipe her face with a clean diaper. Under his gentle touch, she began to relax a little and leaned her head back so he could more easily assess the damage. There were no cuts there beneath the congealing blood, but a long gash on the top of her head continued to ooze. He packed it with another diaper and bandaged her. "You stay quiet here," Ray comforted, "I'll get some help."

Few cars were on the road that stormy night, but Ray managed to flag down an elderly man and his wife who kindly transported them all, still in shock, to the hospital in Chehalis.

Each was lost in their own thoughts as they waited for Aunt Ted to be sutured. Ray broke the long silence of the hospital waiting room with his prophetic words, "That child has been singled out for some special reason…I don't know what…but I have a gut feeling about him…you mark my words…God's hand hooked Malcolm's sweater on that nail." Ray had never attended church in his life and was a bit of a bounder making his statement out of character and totally unexpected.

Uncle Ray's proclamation was prophetic indeed. Fate projected a momentous and long life for this baby.

Chapter II

His World at War

World War II was raging in Europe when Malcolm graduated from high school. His years in school were packed with success. He was hungry for knowledge and consumed Latin, French, mathematics and the sciences to satisfy his ravenous appetite. The National Honor Society was proud to have him wear their badge. The elite French Club voted him King of Mardi Gras. He was well liked and respected by his classmates who honored him as senior class president and as their yearbook's, *"Man most likely to succeed."*

But these were not times when you could rest on your laurels. The world was engulfed in a war madness that was about to change his naïve existence. He signed up for the ASTP, a government program designed to further educate high IQ achievers like Malcolm. This goal was lofty and as carefully thought out as any coming out of Washington, DC, but politics and reality seldom match up. This Army Specialized Training Program was no exception.

The program became a victim of military demands and when he turned eighteen he was shipped out of the University of Utah to Fort Bragg, North Carolina for infantry basic training. His polish and studiousness overqualified him for the job of dog soldier, bayonet training, however, was far above his capability. Street fighter New York buck sergeants tried to teach him to grunt with ferocity and thrust his readied bayonet into a scarecrow enemy soldier. He mimicked the motions, but was finding it impossible to get mad at anyone except the overbearing, in-your-face sergeants.

His staging area enroute to Fort Bragg was Fort Lewis, Washington. While there, he was assigned to Sgtl. Dan Williamson, a quiet, freckle-faced career soldier who was in charge of the movie theater. Malcolm's duties included policing the theater and running the projector. He was conscientious and learned quickly. Dan wanted him to stay and said he could get him transferred to Special Services permanently. As added inducement, he pointed out that he could avoid serving as a rifleman and stay out of harm's way.

Dan subsequently invited him to his home just off the post to meet his folks and stay the weekend. Malcolm enjoyed some welcome home cooking and found Dan's sister and family to be very hospitable. He and Dan shared an upstairs bedroom. It was there that he was shocked to learn that Dan was homosexual. Malcolm wanted no part of that and requested an immediate transfer from his Special Services assignment. That surprising and most unacceptable experience opened his eyes to the fact that men like Dan existed. Malcolm was an off-the-chart heterosexual who cherished women and was so physically attracted to them that he found it impossible to envision a man being attracted to another man.

The dehumanizing rigors of basic training prepared him for what was to follow, but never hardened his soul. He would become a crafty adversary, but never embraced the killer instinct of a true soldier. His performance was exemplary, however, and he graduated from Fort Bragg as a Pfc. Asst. Squad Leader in 1st Platoon, Co. E of the 100th Division. He was a tiny cog in a very big machine for the first time in his life. He went into survival mode.

He was in the PX one day just before he shipped out of Fort Lewis. Coincidentally, a mother and father and their teenaged daughter were there too. The parents, who happened to be from his home town of Eugene, Oregon talked to him thanking him for his service to his country. Their attractive daughter, Beverly, asked if she could write to him overseas. Surprised and honored by her innocently offered request, he gave her his name and Fort Bragg address. Unbeknownst to him, she later visited his parents in Eugene and they became fast friends. She was a comfort to his mother and vice versa. Beverly had felt an instant and strong connection to Emma's handsome son. The letters she wrote almost daily were entertaining, cheerful and decorated with elaborate cartoons. She was an accomplished artist with distinctive, flawless penmanship. As time went on he was teased relentlessly at mail time by those who envied him.

"Here's another love letter for Malcolm," the Sergeant shouted out for all to hear, "He gets more mail from home than any of us. He must be quite a stud!"

Sgt. Erickson was unmerciful with his sarcastic comments and always used McKenna's first name to place emphasis on his abundant mail deliveries rather than the curt last name announcements he usually called out. Malcolm was reluctant, under these circumstances, to admit that he had met this doting female in passing at the PX. To them, it was a hot romance and she became his lover. In his buttoned shirt pocket, he carried her picture inside the metal clad New Testament that she had sent.

When he returned to Eugene after the war, Beverly was ready to continue what she thought of as a two year "engagement." To Malcolm, they were actually just meeting for the first time. He found her to be an attractive and nice girl, the kind you want to take home to meet the folks. That would not be necessary in this case because they already knew her much better than he did. The war had turned his world upside down in many ways.

His education had been interrupted which may have been a blessing in disguise. He had endured a fast-track maturity and was ready for the adult confusing world he now found himself immersed in. He would also benefit from the GI education bill that congress passed at the close of the war. He was entitled to four years of tuition and a small allowance for books. He knew he was going to start college in the fall at the University of Oregon in Eugene. He didn't know what his major would be and that blank had to be filled in on his entrance application. He considered chemistry and the sciences, but the idea of working in a laboratory didn't appeal to him. He liked people and saw himself dealing with them in some way. "Science + People = Doctor" was the simple equation he zeroed in on. He had had no family doctor or other exposure to medicine so this was a non-emotional process of elimination. He filled in the major blank with the words "pre-med." He thought he could change it later if he didn't like the fit. He saved his GI benefit for medical school where costs would be substantially higher. He knew he could live at home in Eugene for the pre-med years. An empathetic counselor provided by the military to help rehabilitation ----------------------- questioned that decision.

"What if you don't get into medical school? The standards are very high and the competition is fierce," he said knowing that the sudden influx of returning soldiers increased the probability of non-acceptance.

"If I still like it by then I'll get in because I always finish what I start," Malcolm stated confidently.

A smile slid across the counselor's face, "Good for you, Malcolm. With that attitude I'm sure you will."

That was 1946 and we need to fill in the preceding two years. His unit shipped out of New York bound for Marseille, France in 1944. Strewn with sunken ships, the French harbor was impassable. They were forced to climb over the side of their ship on rope ladders and were then transported to land in 30-man lifeboats. For the first time it hit home that they were in the war zone because of this ghostly eerie destruction. Ship's masts protruded from the oily water wherever Malcolm looked. The solid ground underfoot was welcome relief from the long and dangerous voyage. German submarines were prevalent in the Atlantic preying on American convoys. This beachhead had been secured within the last few days but their encampment was reportedly safe from enemy artillery. They were warned not to go into the city because friendly French Moroccan soldiers were stabbing Americans whom they could not differentiate, in the dark, from the German enemy.

It took four days to off-load heavy equipment and then they walked north, single file, on either side of the road. Trucks, jeeps and tanks filled the center lane bumper to bumper. Malcolm carried his share of heavy equipment in, including a 75-pound back pack, webb belt with grenades, ammo and canteen and his shoulder-slung M1 rifle. That rifle would be his constant companion and protector. He was young and physically strong from months of general conditioning which lightened his load somewhat. As he marched day after day into oblivion, his thoughts were centered around happier times. Home in Oregon and his beloved McKenzie River. It did not enter his mind that he might never see those things again. The front line, with its smell of gunpowder and death, was a few days ahead. They marched northeast toward the southern most border of the front. The Americans had dug in for the winter near the Maginot Line and the Swiss border. The 100th Division was to replace a unit there that had fought in North Africa and was battle weary. When Malcolm looked into the faces of those men as they marched through, on their way out, he was overcome with emotion. They were vacant shells. Their glazed eyes stared straight ahead as if every inch of humanity had been wrung out of them. He didn't want that to happen to him. He would rather be dead than walk among the living dead. He resolved that he would fly fish on the McKenzie everyday when he returned home to see past what was about to happen. His mother had sent him a postcard of his beloved river that he carried with his metal-covered Bible. The inscription on it read, "May this keep you safe from harm."

The serenity of the Alder forest surrounding his first foxhole was soon broken by a barrage of artillery shells. The distant boom and then the whistling sounds as they passed over had become a daily, and sometimes hourly, reminder that the enemy was just over the hill. He learned to crouch low when he heard that same boom because the shells that struck the closest did not whistle a warning. The ever present threat of enemy soldiers attacking through the woods, especially at night, prompted constant awareness even in sleep.

A few weeks later when they were ordered to move forward on the attack it was almost a relief. Malcolm consciously blotted out the bloody reality of battle and chose instead to remember the miraculous incidents of survival. He had a sixth sense that always put him in the right place at the right time. He read the enemy like he read the wily trout on the McKenzie.

Snow blanketed the Maginot Line on New Year's Eve 1944. Most of the 7th Army, including Patton, was pulled up north to the Battle of the Bulge. E Co. of the 100th Division was left to guard the flank of the southern front. Malcolm's squad leader, S/Sgt. Weirstahl had been wounded two weeks earlier. Buck Sgt. Everly was now in command and Pfc. McKenna took Everly's position. Their squad was assigned a pill box with instructions to hold at any cost against an expected counter attack. McKenna and Sgt. Everly discussed strategy.

"I think we should all be in the bunker here, where it's warmer and protected from artillery fire," Everly announced with as much authority as he could muster. McKenna had always thought Everly was unfit to be their leader. Again, he saw signs of his cowardice.

"You and the rest of the squad stay in there with Profitt and his machine gun," McKenna stated flatly. "I'll take Smitty with me," he gestured toward the road directly below the pill box, "OK?"

McKenna feared the cold a lot less than he feared the Germans. He anticipated they would come marching up the road and wanted to stop them before they reached this valuable bunker. The Maginot Line, a series of concrete fortifications, hadn't done the French much good.

"Fine with me, but aren't you going to be totally exposed down there?" Everly's cowardice was showing again.

"I'll keep my head down. Come on Smitty, let's go." McKenna trusted Smitty who, at 36, was the oldest man in the squad. He was from the Kentucky hills and a crack shot.

The hole was long and deep with plenty of room for two. With a

Shelterhalf pulled over the back side it was surprisingly warm down there.

"You get some sleep, Smitty. I'll take first watch."

Smitty sat with his back against the dirt wall, his knees drawn up for comfort and warmth. He was worn out from the day's long march and was asleep almost instantly.

The moon was full. It reflected off the broad expanse of white snow turning night into dawn. Malcolm looked at his watch to be sure it wasn't midnight yet. He read 11:35 on the luminous dial. New Year's Day 1945, only minutes away. He thought back to this moment a year ago. He was home for the holidays and would report to Fort Lewis in January. Sadness had filled the room. His sister escaped to the kitchen and returned with four glasses and a bottle of chilled champagne. At five minutes to midnight his father stood up and ceremoniously popped the cork. He filled the waiting flutes. His hands were visibly shaking and for once in his life he was speechless. Malcolm knew it was up to him to find something positive to say.

"Here's to the New Year," he said with forced cheerfulness. "I'm looking forward to the adventure it brings."

He looked from his mother's sad eyes to his father's obvious misery.

"Your love has prepared me well and will protect me always."

His confidence was real and they were quick to embrace his heartfelt resolve. He had never let them down and he didn't plan to start now.

Scotty raised his glass to his only son, "Let's drink to a quick and victorious end to this war and your safe homecoming."

* * *

As he crouched there, in his foxhole, his thoughts turned to deer hunting in eastern Oregon. He had a great respect for Native American culture and their way of hunting. He had mastered the art of bow hunting and silently stalking his prey. Often times evening hunts would carry over into sudden darkness and then moonlight. He loved that quiet time and the nocturnal sounds that painted such vivid pictures.

Now he was thousands of miles away, in France, hidden and stalking people, not deer, in the revealing moonlight. It was midnight but he heard no bells. He was suddenly lonely and felt tears freezing on his unshaven cheeks. He pulled his right hand from his warm pocket and raised it with an imaginary glass of champagne.

"Here's to happy people and sanity…may this madness end soon."

New Year's was ushered in with strange sounds carried astonishingly unaltered with the cold night air. The distinct creaking of wagon wheels pulled along by horses over icy roads told him that the Germans were moving in their direction. Gas shortages had forced them to resort, in desperation, to primitive methods, but they were able to counterattack despite the setbacks. He waited and watched the road intently. The Germans were like the cardboard cutouts at the practice range as they came up the road and over an ice-encrusted ridge in the distance. They were perfect black silhouettes against the whiteness of the snow. McKenna nudged Smitty with his foot.

"They're here…get up," he whispered.

As he had predicted, the Germans attention was on the pill box on the hillside to their left. They were like sitting ducks exposed to the firepower of McKenna and Smitty. They must have thought the American Army was coming up the road to attack them. Had they known that the army was two lone men they could have easily overrun them. They retreated. It was later revealed that a whole regiment was counter attacking that night. They had no idea that the American force consisted of one company and, in reality, two men dug in along the road. A deer hunter, fighting Indian-style, had pulled off a spectacular bluff.

The Maginot Line was curved around the high ground of a hill at the point where Co. E was defending. Malcolm's squad was at the extreme left flank. The attacking German regiment had been thwarted by that remaining emplacement, but in the process one whole platoon was taken prisoner and many men were killed. Word came down after the war that many of those captured had died of malnutrition and tuberculosis. Malcolm's guardian angel had seen to it that he was in the exact spot to become a hero and to, once again, survive.

* * *

When the company regrouped after the battle, Buck Sgt. Everly suddenly became incoherent. He walked in circles and fell into a shell hole. He got up covered with mud and shouted, "Blood must flow in the streets of Berlin….Victory is at hand…" He was taken by the medics back to the hospital and was never seen again. Malcolm received the Bronze Star, a promotion to Staff Sergeant and was now the squad leader. He would lead his squad through many more, equally harrowing, battles before the war ended.

Again the Division found itself fanned out across an open field moving forward to a German village. This time a hilltop farmhouse ahead allowed the enemy to direct deadly artillery fire. McKenna flattened in the wheat stubble, his heart pounding, was protected from the shrapnel whirring overhead. The incessant whistling of the shells was unnerving. A lull afforded him the opportunity to get to his feet and motion his squad forward. They ran until their mouths were dry and they had no breath left. Flattened on the ground once again, they rested a few moments and then repeated their advance until they reached a protected area at the base of the hill where the farmhouse stood. The attack had become a "V" with McKenna's squad at it's' point. He knew instinctively that the safest place to be under heavy, well directed, artillery fire was as far forward as you could get. His squad suffered no casualties. A machine gun emplacement in that farmhouse was straffing the hill above them. They were ordered by radio to retreat to a deep ravine down hill on the right flank of the advance. The battalion commander, Col. Edwards, had been watching with his binoculars from a safe haven. He wanted to talk to the Sergeant who was leading the charge. As soon as McKenna jumped into the ravine he was ordered to report to the command post.

"What's your name, Sergeant?"

"McKenna, Sir." He had not been that close to a battalion commander before. In fact, the company commander was rarely seen.

"You were up there alone. What did you see? What do you think about a frontal assault on that hill?" Col. Edwards was showing this lowly Sergeant a great deal of respect.

"Sir, if you want my honest opinion it cannot be done that way without unacceptable casualties," McKenna leveled his gaze directly into Col. Edwards eyes.

"What would you have me do then?" Edwards challenged the baby-faced McKenna.

"If you have access to artillery, I would bombard that vulnerable farmhouse through the night and attack at dawn," McKenna's response was immediate and to the point.

"Thanks, Sergeant. Go back and get some rest now…you'll need it," Edwards said respectfully. In McKenna's experience this was an unheard of conversation in the heat of battle. McKenna and Edwards would never meet again.

All night long artillery shells whistled overhead and exploded on the hilltop. The next morning they walked up the hill and on through the sleepy village of Sierstahl. No shots were fired. A fat, hysterical civilian ran down the walkway from his house and confronted the approaching McKenna. Malcolm was caught by surprise when the irate man lunged forward at him. He was eyeball to eyeball with a madman and plunged his 45 deep into that soft belly. He had every right to pull the trigger. He didn't. The old German ran off like a frightened rabbit and McKenna walked on, satisfied that when the war was over he would have no regrets. He would forget the absurdity of war but benefit from the honing of his survival instincts. He would discover that life is a war of a different kind.

A few months later the German army collapsed. Their country was rotten at its core. Their supreme leader was a madman. They were destined to fail from the moment they aroused the sleeping giant, the United States.

Chapter III

The Long Wait

The 100th Division was stationed at a barracks on the outskirts of Fortzheim after the war's end. This was an unbelievable military post built of stone with luxurious embellishments. Hitler wanted his elite SS troops stationed there in order to experience the best accommodations possible. The Americans coming directly from the grime of war thought they were in heaven. They relaxed into this cushion of soft life they had not seen before. This was a military Hilton. German employees took care of all the laundry and kitchen facilities. There was no scutwork duty like KP. McKenna suddenly realized that as a staff Sergeant he was being treated with great respect. He had a private room and ate at a table in the officer's special dining room. A squad leader has more men under his direct control that any officer and he had developed such a close relationship with his men that he was uncomfortable with this arrangement.

Going home was on everyone's mind. The wait would be prolonged indefinitely because there were so many soldiers in Europe that ships to carry them across the Atlantic were at a premium. A point system was devised to put the most deserving at the top of the list of returnees. Five points were given for medals earned such as the Combat Infantry Badge, Purple Heart and Bronze or Silver Stars. Points were also awarded for each month served overseas. McKenna ended up with 85 points under that system. His wait was almost eight months whereas most of the troops waited over a year.

To help make this void more palatable, two-week trips to Paris and the Riviera were handed out on a rotating basis. A surprising number of soldiers were so pleased with the GI Hilton that they ignored these side trips. McKenna, however, reveled in such opportunity and was more than happy to travel. The warm sunshine on the French Riviera beckoned and he took several train trips out of the cold to Nice.

He stayed at the lavish Negresco Hotel where he would awaken to breakfast in bed. This world of opulence was so opposite to what he had experienced just weeks earlier that he was uneasy. There was no struggle for survival here so he turned his attention to another basic instinct.

The only training he had received in the army to prepare him for this playground was a single government poster. A grim-faced Uncle Sam pointing an accusing finger warned of a serendipitous enemy as vicious as the German army. It was called VD. Malcolm would not have to fear this enemy because of his laughable naiveté with women. His attraction to the opposite sex was strong, but he saw women as untouchable works of art. He had not learned how to break them down and examine the working parts like he had his M1 rifle. He was about to learn how animate and available these French coquettes really were.

The first morning of his vacation he went to the PX. His ration card allowed him to buy chocolate bars and cigarettes. He was still a non-smoker in spite of his front line, gut level survival. Everyone around him lit up to calm their nerves. They thought it weird that he didn't do the same and continually offered him cigarettes. He always refused.

"You may be dead within the hour, you need to enjoy yourself more," they pleaded continually.

"I don't need smoke in my lungs to relax. I need lots of oxygen," Malcolm's quick logic foretold that he would likely always be misunderstood and envied.

Malcolm's cigarettes and chocolate would be barter material. The civilians in Nice could not get them in their markets. A carton of cigarettes that he could buy for one dollar went for twenty-five dollars on the barter system. If for no other reason than the obvious monetary advantages, he was glad that he had never taken up the habit. As he walked down the crowded line along the counter picking out items, he overheard two girls talking in French.

"Il est un mignon gars," the big-eyed brunette giggled to her friend while nodding in McKenna's direction.

He was thinking the same about her. Thanks to Miss Blais' French class he understood her comment. She had not anticipated that he had studied Latin and French in high school. He walked through the line and then stopped at a counter near the windows pretending to organize his wallet as he replaced his ration card. He watched the eager GIs, who had come in expressly to engage the girls in conversation, hover around them. After the procession thinned and they all walked away disappointed, he walked directly to her section of the counter.

"Je parle un peu de Francais," he smiled knowingly.

She was delighted that he knew what she had said to her girlfriend. They small-talked and he invited her to the USO dance that night.

He anxiously waited in the lobby rehearsing bits of conversation and hoping his inexperience would not offend her. She walked confidently into the room and cast a devastating smile in his direction. She was even more beautiful than he remembered. High heels, short black dress and white fur jacket turned all heads in her direction. Her big dark eyes and pixie features reminded him of Betty Boop, the cartoon vamp.

She ignored all the admiring eyes riveted on her and walked up to him with her small hands extended invitingly. He was about to take one and kiss it gallantly, as seemed befitting to the princess she was, but she did not stop. She encircled him in fur, caressing his neck and planted a warm kiss on his cheek. He was speechless as she took his arm and they followed the music into the dance hall. The hoard of homesick GIs standing against the walls were dumb struck and the first small seeds on the trail of envy had been planted.

The long train ride back to Fortzheim allowed plenty of time for Malcolm to daydream about the war. He wanted to remember the humane and not the horror of it. He thought about birth and death. He thought about the day the 100th was marching through a nameless German village where civilians were sniping at them from the upstairs windows. On the outskirts as they passed sporadic farmhouses with the ever present barns attached, heavy artillery fire came whistling in from the retreating German army ahead. He motioned his squad off the road and they took cover in one of the nearby barns. The smell and warmth of the manure was welcome relief from the cold and gunfire outside. At first their attention was frozen on the shells bursting all around, spewing deadly shrapnel. The milk cow lying in her stall, close to the back door of the attached house, went unnoticed.

Smitty was the first to see her. "Well, I'll be damned, look over here," his words eased the tension.

Everyone looked in the direction he was pointing to see a mound of cow hair projecting above the straw. A lull in the explosions outside allowed them to hear her moans. She was having a calf right in the middle of all this chaos and destruction. They watched the happy event and when the cow stood up to lick her struggling wet calf, McKenna spoke.

"Life goes on and so do we. Let's get out of here before some kraut finds us in this dead-end trap."

Thinking back, McKenna mused at how close life and death really are in the short time we occupy this earth. He vowed to make good use of every minute of his existence. To pull himself up from this depth of reality he next thought about Christmas.

The French village they had liberated on Christmas Eve surrounded them with the most meaningful joy of this holiday he had ever experienced. His childhood was as happy as two loving parents could make it and Christmas was always special. The smells of turkey and dressing, the family feasts with relatives all around, his father sitting in the kitchen Christmas morning running the mixer of Tom and Jerry batter. How red his cheeks would glow after all his friends had come and gone. Yes, Christmas brings out the best in all of us and that Christmas, in that small French village ravaged by war and then suddenly liberated, was a once in a lifetime event. Malcolm lived "Joy to the World" that night. There was no turkey or pumpkin pie, but a long table was set with his men all around. He would never forget their tired, beaming faces. He was so close to them and owed his life to them. They felt the kinship too and trusted his judgment to bring them through this gauntlet of death.

Their grateful host had brought out an armload of vintage wine. He had somehow managed to hide it from the occupying Nazi army. He filled the glasses all around and held his own high to say two French words they could all understand, "Pour Noel." Those sincere words coming from that happy man would be burned into McKenna's brain forever.

The train lurched to a stop and his arrival back to Fortzheim and reality turned his attention to his new assignment. The order had arrived before he left for the Riviera. He was to become the military mayor of Langenalb, Germany. His squad would man a road block to protect the towns from the marauding French army bent on retribution.

They were billeted in a tall corner house with sixteen steps leading up to the front entry. This was significant because heavy boxes of K-rations had to be shouldered and carried up. McKenna slipped on those steep steps and fell to the bottom, rations and all. He was unable to get on his feet because his right ankle had been severely injured. The hausfrau, Hilda, ran out and picked him up bodily as if he were a child. She ascended those steep steps with ease and placed him gently on the couch. She was typical of the sturdy German farm women. McKenna was somewhat chagrined by such a rescue and was glad his men were not around at the time to witness the event. The thought crossed his mind of the groom being carried across the threshold by his bride. He smiled to himself in spite of it all.

Hilda mothered these American intruders in an amazingly impersonal way. She cooked and did their laundry. She poulticed McKenna's ankle with some unknown smelly ointment. The men all agreed it was manure. It seemed to work in spite of the unpleasant aroma. They teased Malcolm about his new protector and girlfriend.

Langenalb was on the edge of the Black Forest near a former hunting preserve for the elite SS troops. None of the townspeople were allowed to have guns, by decree, even after the war. McKenna was anxious to explore that area thinking that fresh meat would be a welcome change from the monotonous K-rations. He followed a tiny creek across the meadows leading to the woods. He dropped a grasshopper into the clear water and was surprised to see a 12-inch, brown trout come out from under the mossy edge and devour it. He had free-time because his men were drawing guard duty and he was the omnipotent mayor of the city. This was a dramatic change from his usual participation.

Fishing and hunting were his first love and now his men needed meat. He was obligated to bring home the bacon, so to speak. He accepted the challenge happily. He used the proverbial safety pin, string and willow pole with grasshopper bait to catch 22 beautiful trout that day. The mostly foot-wide stream surprisingly held unsuspected bounty. He doubted anyone had ever fished there. His men were eagerly looking forward to the feast of fried trout that night. Their spirits fell, however, when Hilda brought three bowls of curled up, pale, boiled fish to the table. No one dreamed she would need to be instructed on how to fry a trout. They ate them good-naturedly so as not to offend the cook. In truth, even those mutilated fish were a welcome relief from rations.

From the head of the table, McKenna, whose glorious feat was somewhat diluted with boiling water made an announcement. "While I was out I explored the edge of those woods today. There are deer and wild boar signs. How does venison sound?" He smiled and added, "I'll see to it that Hilda knows how to use the oven."

"I love to hunt," Smitty volunteered.

"I went rabbit hunting a few times," Sam, an Alabama native, added helpfully.

"Alright then, it's settled. The three of us will go on a meat hunt tomorrow. To make it more interesting why don't we each put ten dollars in the pot? The one who brings the most meat to the table wins the prize," McKenna challenged confidently.

"I'd like to come as an observer," Vince, the medic, who never carried a gun, welcomed the chance to share a new adventure. He liked to stay close to McKenna for whom he had great respect. Vince was nearest to Smitty in age. The late 30s made them the "old men" of the squad. Vince was always intrigued by the dynamics of McKenna's unwavering, effortless control over his men in spite of the fact that he was the youngest. He was still a teenager at 19 and had grown a little moustache as proof that he was actually old enough to shave.

The three hunters separated at the edge of the woods. Vince stayed with McKenna. The dense forest was checker-boarded with narrow dirt roads spaced about a mile apart. McKenna surmised that a privileged few hunters would take a stand and drivers with dogs would come from a distance and run the deer past them. This suspicion was born out when he found a tree stand a few miles from their starting point. It consisted of a rustic 20-foot ladder made of tree limbs secured to a tall tree. A one-man floored and railed nest was built into the crook of the tree at the top of the ladder.

"I'm going to climb up there and wait until dark if I have to," he informed Vince who had never hunted and was already in the dark about what was going on.

"I'll sit quietly with the ladder as a back rest here on the ground. Is that okay?"

"It may be a few hours and I don't want you to move or make a sound. Understood?" McKenna feared that Vince's inexperience would spoil his well-conceived plan.

"I got it. You won't hear a sound down here," he reassured McKenna who was halfway up the ladder already. He just had room to sit cross-legged with his M1 resting over the railing for comfort during the long wait and for a steady aim if a deer should appear.

Smitty and Sam went tramping through the woods in opposite directions. They figured that the more territory they could cover the better chance they would have of surprising a deer in it's' bed. They thought they heard animals running ahead, but never got a clear shot in the dense underbrush. Two hours of fighting the thicket convinced them that a cold beer back in town sounded like a better idea than chasing phantoms. They returned to the house a full hour before sunset.

"McKenna is the most persistent S.O.B. I've ever met. He'll stay out 'til midnight I suppose," Sam laughed as he soothed his parched throat with a long swallow of cold beer. "Those Scots will do anything for twenty bucks."

"All he has to do is get one buck for our twenty bucks and if he sees one out there it's his for sure. He's the best shot I've ever seen," Smitty replied.

McKenna and Vince waited patiently. It was dusk when a small deer appeared far down the road. It was eating the tall grass and unaware of McKenna high up in the tree stand. He adjusted his open sight for the distance, took careful aim and squeezed the trigger. The loud report startled Vince who was half asleep.

"Did you hit it?"

"I don't know, it's too far away. I saw it jump into the air," he called excitedly as he began his descent. "I'm coming down." They walked to the kill and paced the distance of 630 feet, a very long shot with an open sight in poor light. It was a whrey three point, about the size of a large dog. They tied its feet over a long pole and carried it back together.

Vince complimented him as they walked through the meadow, "That was a long shot and you hit it high in the front shoulder. Very impressive… it was a clean kill."

"I was lucky. They say you always hunt better when you're hungry and we need the fresh meat." McKenna saved those little antlers and took them home as a souvenir. On the wall next to his mule deer and elk they would be laughable in size, but gigantic in memory.

Their assignment in Langenalb ended two weeks later. They would miss Hilda and the grateful people of that little farm town. McKenna would miss the unusual hunting and fishing experiences.

* * *

He took the next available Riviera trip. He could not get Blanche, his Betty Boop girl, out of his mind. He hurried to the PX to see her but she was not there. He was told that her grandmother was seriously ill and she had returned home to Lyon. He walked along the beach not feeling the warm sun or seeing the beauty of it all. This was no longer a happy place and his thoughts returned home. He was suddenly bitter about the long wait. There must be room on one of those ships for him. The last report he had heard was that it would be at least another year. Beverly's letters were a constant reminder of that far away haven. She had been so faithful to write almost daily. He would get groups of three or four letters at a time. He enjoyed them more when he was on the front line. Now they only rubbed salt in his homesickness wound.

He looked out across the blue expanse of the Mediterranean. Home was out there somewhere. His gaze shifted to the beach and a bikini-clad young female lying there alone. He approached her, blocking the sun to get her attention.

"You look as alone as I feel….are you?"

Looking up into the handsome GI's face, the pretty young French girl giggled. "Yes, I am alone. Please sit down here and talk to me. I want to practice the English."

"Your English is great, but I could use some help with my very inadequate French," he was glad to have such an excuse to befriend this charming little French emissary.

She was too young to be a raving beauty like Blanche, but she was cute. Her vivacious personality more than made up for the lack of certain physical attributes that maturity brings to a woman. Her dark, flawless skin and the sweet perfection of her face were more than enough femininity to hold his attention. She seemed a perfect match for his limited understanding of women. Her name was Evelyn.

They laughed together all during his ten day stay in Nice. She introduced him to her aunt who was well placed in the undercover exchange market. She would pay him the black market price for American cigarettes and chocolate. Then they would go out on the town with the proceeds and buy one dollar steak sandwiches for an inflated ten dollars. (The uncut meat had U.S. Army stamped on it). He could afford the best champagne and one night as he walked her home he was showing the effects of that special treat. He rarely drank so that it didn't take much to affect him. She used the word *zig zag* in her casual French. He confused that with *zig zig*. This lingual mix up led to a comical scene because the first means *drunk* and the second, *let's make love*.

He forgot all about Blanche and home. On the day before he was to depart, Evelyn introduced him to her cousin Blaise whom they had run into accidentally. He found himself looking into the biggest, greenest eyes he had ever seen. He was mesmerized instantly and barely heard her invitation.

"I want to show you my modeling posters." Blaise was a professional model, a natural consequence of her classic beauty. She had all the maturity that Evelyn lacked.

Evelyn said she was expected home and left them alone. She would meet him later that night. Blaise then put her arm around McKenna and led him to her apartment. The warmth of her mink jacket pressing so close was carrying him to other places. Was this a dream?

When they entered her luxurious apartment it looked very real to him. Pictures of her adorned the walls. They were very Hollywood, very glamorous. Every state of dress and undress was portrayed. She was almost as captivating on the wall as she was standing there right next to him. He could not shake the feeling that he had been transported from the real world. He was in no way prepared for what she did next. She left the room and came back with a very old man.

"This is my grandfather, Dee." She was holding tight to the senile character with transparent skin. He could barely stand. She helped him into a chair.

"I'll get some coffee," she said as she departed to the kitchen. Dee could not speak English and was deaf so he and McKenna just stared awkwardly at each other until Blaise returned with their coffee.

"He has nowhere to go so I take care of him," she explained.

McKenna thought she was the most unlikely nursemaid he could ever imagine. He was even more shocked when she sat on Dee's lap and caressed his wrinkled face. She smoothed his wispy hair and kissed him on the cheek.

"Je vous amour," she purred in his ear.

This display of affection was so warm and unexpected that McKenna found himself envying the old man, "I hope I have someone like you around when I get old."

"You will," she smiled warmly. "You have such a kind heart. Evelyn has told me all about you."

Blaise's directness was as disarming as her beauty. McKenna was sorry now that he would not get to stay in Nice indefinitely. This was a complete turnaround from the feeling he had when he arrived a week earlier. What a difference the spell of the great feminine makes on a man and he had not yet realized that the greatest surprise was yet to come.

Blaise took the old man back to his room and when she returned she sat on McKenna's lap. Her kisses were warm and lingering and she led him willingly into an evening of unexpected, all-consuming amour.

* * *

Once again, on the long train ride back to Germany he had considerable time to relive the past. He thought about some close calls he had suffered on the front line. There were three rifle bullet near misses. A hole in his back pack and one in his helmet were proof of that. The spent bullet that penetrated the exterior of his helmet yet failed to enter the interior lining was the most disturbing. That bullet went round and round between the layers sounding like a mad hornet. He didn't know what was going on at first and threw his helmet to the ground in a state of panic. When he discovered the cause he marveled at the fact that the rifleman firing that shot was a sharp shooter indeed, but luckily was just far enough away.

He did receive one shrapnel wound and subsequently was honored with the Purple Heart. Again he was protected from serious injury, this time by layers of winter clothing. The nickel-sized metal fragment barely penetrated his parka and created a severe bruise and superficial laceration on his left forearm. He sought treatment a few days later because it became badly infected. He wondered why he had been so lucky when so many around him had been killed or sent to the hospital with serious wounds. He thought about what his Uncle Ray had said many years before. He had a destiny that must be fulfilled. He wondered what it would be. The way things were shaping up he suspected it must be extremely important.

He tried to think of some lighter moments to clear his head of these grim thoughts. He remembered how surprised he was to hear his name called out when they were marching along that road into Germany a few miles behind Patton's tanks. It was several days after Easter Sunday and the Germans were retreating so fast it was grueling to keep up as a foot soldier. An artillery unit was coming through and someone was calling his name from a truck. It drove alongside and he held up his hand not imagining anyone in this maze of soldiers would know his name.

"So, you're Sgt. McKenna. I knew this was the 100th Division and hoped to find you," the Lieutenant handed McKenna a small, black diary. "I found this in a house we stayed in a few hundred miles back. It's so touching I felt obligated to return it to you. You should be a writer when we get back."

McKenna had been heartsick when he realized he had left his beloved diary on the window sill near the kitchen table in the house they had searched on Easter Sunday. He was certain it was lost for good. He could still smell the roast beef that had been left in the oven by the fleeing

Germans. His squad had eaten that magnificent Easter dinner at the family's kitchen table. He had written in his diary to note their good fortune and then had forgotten to retrieve it from the window sill when they had hurriedly vacated the house. It was truly a miracle he thought now as he returned it to his breast pocket where it had always been safe from the harsh elements. Maybe, like the Lieutenant said, he should be a writer.

DIARY NOTES
He was still thinking about his destiny and what he would do when he got home when the train arrived in Fortzheim. His private room and royal treatment there were not enough to keep him from resenting the fact that he should be home now. He was tired of this army life. He never had adjusted to regimentation.

Orders came down that he was to take his squad on 4:00am raids of individual German houses. He was to look for firearms or any evidence of German soldiers being sheltered. Civilians were already angry at the Americans and these forays only added to their distrust. Herding shocked, sleepy night-shirted people around was not McKenna's idea of fun. He abruptly changed his mind on one such raid when a tall, slender very blue-eyed, blonde victim looked him in the eye. That look said, "I am at your mercy, please be nice to me."

He felt like the pirate, Bluebeard, he had read so much about. He knew she was taking advantage of the situation and acting out her fantasy and he suddenly wanted to act out his. The instant attraction to her was overwhelming.

He scribbled a note on a sheet of paper at a nearby desk. It read: "You are hereby ordered to appear at the town square under the clock at 8:00pm tonight for further questioning."

He arrived there at 7:45 hoping she could read English. She dutifully arrived at 8:00 and in perfect English greeted him, "I was taught to always cooperate with the police."

"I'm not the police and I really don't have much authority over you. I hope you understand that," he confessed.

She took his hand in hers, "I know, but in the midst of all this horror you seemed like a beacon of hope. I had to come."

They dated regularly until he shipped out three months later. He never dreamed he would be so reluctant to leave Fortzheim.

The train trip to Brest, France was long and lonely. He could not get

Frieda out of his mind. She was stately and strong, yet feminine in every way. When they were together all the confusion around them evaporated and their opposite worlds fused together. Now he was leaving the familiar and heading for the unknown once again…home.

Chapter IV

Almost Home

The vessel they boarded in Brest was a converted Liberty ship, ironically built at Kaiser Shipyards in Portland, Oregon. The whole scenario about women taking over for the men, all off to war comes to play. Rosie the Riveter was born and would go down in history. He would be grateful that Rosie's rivets were well placed before the 21-day nightmare was over.

The usual timeframe for the North Atlantic crossing was one week, but a hurricane changed all that. A Liberty ship was converted to a troupe carrier by lining the hold with endless bunks. These beds were simple affairs, chain-held shelves three-feet apart with four-inch mattresses. Over 400 GIs could be stored below on this most utilitarian crossing.

The propeller sounds vibrated throughout the ship and foretold the magnitude of the storm outside. They emitted a laboring groan climbing the 60-foot waves. When the ship was falling into the valley between waves those same props spun helplessly in mid-air and the deafening vibration gave the distinct feeling that the ship was breaking in half. The hurricane precluded opening the hatches. McKenna sat on his duffle bag, propped up against the wall and stared at the riveted metal walls for hours at a time. He wondered when they would pop out and fill the room with flying missiles as sea water came rushing in. Most were so sick they could not enjoy this pastime. Sea sickness became contagious when vomit from the upper bunks rained down on the unsuspecting victims below. When the storm was at its peak, the upper bunk chains twisting and grinding against the bed frames, both mattresses and men were dumped to the ground. Most sat helpless and green-tinged, praying to step foot on land…any land would do. Much as they longed for home they would have been more than happy to return to France.

McKenna told himself that sea sickness was just a state of mind. He made himself believe that if he kept something in his stomach, he could avoid its deadly throws. He pulled himself up the stairs to the mess hall by gripping the hand rail with such a sense of purpose that he became a part of the ship. After a few days he was all alone in this endeavor. He sat in the now empty mess hall with his legs wrapped around the crossed pipe table base for stability. He even managed a smile as he watched the plastic cups; plates and bowls slide from one end of the long table to the other. He thought of the cocoon of the earthen foxholes back in Germany. Even that seemed like a paradise to him now. He was glad he hadn't joined the navy.

Little did he know that this 21-day crossing of the Atlantic was an aberration. It was not routine and they truly had been in danger of sinking. When the ship finally reached New York it was stripped of all its' lifeboats and superstructure. Eight crewmembers had suffered severe injuries. That ship was doomed to never sail again. This battle with the North Atlantic combined with all those near misses in Europe and the many yet to come, added credence to the fact that McKenna led a charmed life indeed.

The trans-continental train trip from New York to Fort Lewis, Washington was uneventful and the clicking sound of the wheels on solid rails was a welcome sound to the weary traveler. The mustering out routine there was tedious and anti-climactic. He was so close and yet still so far away from home. It was one final army-sponsored *hurry up and wait* episode and ingrained in him the feeling that his destiny would happily begin when he was finally discharged.

The 300 mile train ride south to Eugene was slow, but made tolerable by the fact that he was now back in familiar territory at last. He was glued to the window, fascinated that the world out here had not changed at all. His folks knew that he was in Fort Lewis but had no idea when he would come home. He wanted it that way and cringed at the thought of a gathering in the train station. He would not know how to handle that embarrassment. He got off the train in his dress uniform with duffel bag slung over his shoulder. He stood there staring at the white station sign… *Eugene*…as the train departed in a cloud of steam behind him. He looked to the left at the open doors marked, *Railway Express*. He thought back to all those times he had gotten off his bicycle, after peddling 12 miles from home or school, to pick up a bundle of *San Francisco Chronicle* dailies. He used to ride straight up Willamette Street dropping them off dutifully at the magazine stores. He was paid two dollars a week for that job. His

Uncle Carl worked at the express office too. He could still see him pulling the heavy four-wheel cart loaded with packages and mail. He had met his Uncle there many times after work. They liked to drive up the McKenzie River for evening fishing expeditions. He wondered why Carl did not come out now to retrieve his cart, but then remembered he was now retired.

McKenna turned west and walked down the tracks to Washington Street. He followed Washington toward the Willamette River. Every house he passed was a landmark. Suddenly that quaint neighborhood was illuminated by a bright light from above. He was closing in on the corner house on Jefferson, with the ancient Hawthorne tree that shaded his bedroom window and the familiar brick chimney with its perpetual wood smoke curling lazily skyward. He passed Beau's Market where his mother had cashed all those railroad paychecks which his father worked so hard for. She had then paid the grocery bill, so dutifully itemized and neatly spindled on little yellow sheets. The store-fronted house looked tiny now. How could it ever have been such a hub of activity? The world he was coming back from made his past seem so very quaint. He would never again see it through child-like eyes. It was sad somehow. He suddenly realized that he was not the person who had left here a few short years earlier. Home had not changed; it was he who was not the same. A tear formed in the corner of his eye. He willed it to stop.

He had regained his composure by the time he reached the back door. He knocked for the first time in his life. He wanted his mother, Emma, to greet him there. Slowly the door cracked open and then her arms flew into the air as she screamed, "Malcolm!" and rushed to embrace him. His body felt protective and strong against her wiry thinness. This homecoming was the culmination of her daily prayers. They could not speak, but their embrace spoke volumes and made up for the years of separation.

When his father came home from work another emotional reunion drained the rest of his strength. He was in a cloudlike trance for his meetings with his sister, nearby relatives and friends that evening. He went to bed exhausted and thought about meeting his loyal letter writer, Beverly, the next day. Who was she, really? What was she going to expect from him?

Emma had called the Culps the evening of Malcolm's arrival to warn Beverly that he planned to visit the next day. Her anticipation of that meeting was overpowering. She too had trouble sleeping, but her questions were different than Malcolm's. She truly believed in love at first sight and had experienced it with him there in the PX at Fort Lewis three years earlier. That feeling had not faded for her and, in fact, had grown stronger with each passing day. She believed that she could not possibly feel this way unless it was mutual. His letters had been heartfelt and warm. Her only question was…had the war robbed him of his innocence? The high school graduation picture that she treasured of him showed a pure heart that matched her own. Her parents were salt of the earth, God-fearing Christians and she mirrored those beliefs. She had long ago befriended Malcolm's parents and they could readily accept her as their daughter-in-law. The amazing fact was that they had never uttered a word about Beverly to their son. They waited patiently for him to speak his own feelings. They had always treated him with such respect. His strong feelings of independence and self control had developed because of their confidence in his judgment.

He cautiously knocked on her front door. Beverly opened it with a burst of energy and expectation. She beamed with pure joy. They embraced and he felt pillowy softness against his hard, muscular body. She was Rubinesque in a pleasing way that most men would find extremely sexy. She had a beautiful, kind face and soft, warm hands that he admired as she showed him to the waiting couch. He sat there feeling like an intruder. She sensed his discomfort and hurried to the kitchen to get a tray with two cool drinks. He did not feel ready to talk about the war and so he was conversationally limited. He questioned her about her life and came away feeling he had known her forever. She was easy to talk to in a *girl next door* sort of way. He knew that they would become good friends, but he had no romantic inclinations. This was going to be difficult.

Malcolm was not only confused about Beverly, he was confused about everything. His adventures overseas had left him unsure about the quietness of home. He was still walking on war legs while desperately searching for his peace legs.

He dated Beverly for about six months to make sure that his initial assessment of their future together had been accurate. She was the epitome of the *quietness of home*. She was too nice. When he told her of his true feelings she was heartbroken.

"But we kissed so many times….even while lying on the couch," she lamented.

She expressed her guilt at having committed such an assault on her virginity. To her, kissing was a sin unless you were married. Under these circumstances, Malcolm felt the same and he carried a burden of guilt which only added to his dilemma further. He remained friends with

Beverly and, in fact, they were even closer once she accepted the truth. Two years later she invited him to her wedding.

When he came down the reception line to kiss the bride on her cheek, she whispered, "You were my first and only love."

Chapter V

No Choice

Malcolm was still adjusting to civilian life when he threw himself blindly into college life. Books became his refuge. His study habits were impeccable because he was so focused. He wanted to deny that part of him that cried out for the adventure he had encountered after the war in Europe. Common sense held him in a vice. He knew there was no future in vagabond life, but he couldn't completely shake his need for exploring the world he knew was out there.

While in this confused state he met Beth. She, also, was not grounded. She was working in the office of the local newspaper and living with her mother, Abigail. Abigail was masterfully controlling. Somehow she made Beth feel guilty about everything. An ingrained inferiority complex made her life miserable. She was looking for a way out of that maternal prison. Beth had no desire for further education, but she was instantly attracted to Malcolm's goal oriented approach to life.

Motivated by such mutual need, their chemistry was electric. Static electric when they first touched. They kissed and the world around them disappeared. Time would never change that part of their relationship even though Malcolm's horizons would broaden dramatically and Beth's would not. That changing life perspective would be his to bear alone. She fell deeply in love and would love Malcolm for the rest of her life. His intelligence and daring captivated her completely. She instinctively knew how to express her love physically with him. She was uninhibited.

It was this chemistry that turned Malcolm's head. At this point in time, he badly needed a soft shoulder. Beth was soft all over. She oozed feminine warmth and her kisses made him euphoric. She was his sheltered port in the academic storm. He forgot all about his need for far away adventure. She was close to home and she programmed her schedule to accommodate his. He found himself content with the best of both worlds. His pre-med studies were not challenging enough so he added French, higher math and philosophy. He fought the boredom of hometown life with the excesses his boundless energy demanded…college life for his mind and Beth for his body.

The three years of pre-med passed quickly. He was accepted into medical school as he had expected and predicted confidently to that counselor before the war. He would be moving from home to Portland. What about Beth? He wondered if he could get along without her.

He knew she would be missed and he would have to fill that void with medicine. She deserved someone who could return her devotion. He knew he was not that man. This was the obvious time to end their relationship. He agonized over how to tell her. He knew she would be devastated.

That evening he was seated at his desk studying for an anthropology exam scheduled for the next afternoon. He was concentrating on the task before him, better than he had of late, now that he had finally made the decision to move to Portland without Beth. Suddenly the phone rang. It was an unexpected call from Beth. Her voice was quiet and apologetic. She had been sitting by her phone for over an hour anguishing about whether or not to dial his number.

"Malcolm….I went to the doctor today."

"What happened? Are you sick? You haven't said anything to me about feeling bad," he interrupted with alarm.

"No, I'm fine. A little nauseated that's all, but I'm fine," Beth hesitated again.

Her throat was parched and her heart pounding. She was beginning to feel that this call was a mistake. The last thing she wanted to do was interfere with his concentration in the middle of final exams. She knew she should wait, but this secret was too earth-shaking to hold inside.

"I'm pregnant!" she blurted out excitedly.

Malcolm's thought processes shut down as soon as he heard those words. He felt a sudden empty feeling in his chest. It was as though his heart had stopped beating. Numbness radiated throughout his body. He could not speak.

"Are you there?" the profound silence scared Beth. He was never speechless. He always had quick responses, especially to problems. "Talk to me…I need you to talk to me."

"Beth, that's……great. I'm so relieved you're not ill," he needed time to think. He mumbled something about needing to hit the books. "I'll see you tomorrow when you get off work. You are still working, right?"

"Yes, I'm working. Come by the house on the way home from campus. I'll look forward to your company," Beth tried to reassure him that she had everything under control.

Malcolm closed his books. It was only 9:00pm, but he went to bed. He wanted to close his eyes and sleep to clear his fogged brain. This feeling was new to him. He had lived through many dangers and problems, but this was beyond logic and beyond his control. He pulled his knees up into a fetal position and wept. He cried big tears for the first time in his life. He finally drifted off to restless sleep around midnight. His last thoughts dwelled on what he would do to earn a living for a family. He reasoned he could not go to medical school now. He thought about working in the cannery where he had worked summers to put away money for clothes and books. Maybe his dad could get him a job on the railroad. Tears welled up and flowed down his cheeks once again.

His mother was alarmed when she saw him at the breakfast table the next morning. His eyes were swollen and red. He was not his usual cheerful, buoyant self. He was too quiet. She had never seen him like this.

"Malcolm, are you feeling alright?" she managed to question knowing that he never talked about his problems with her.

She didn't push. She always respected his stoic nature. She knew he wanted it that way. Since his return from the war he had been harboring a deep-seated restlessness. He never spoke about what really happened over there, but it had changed him in ways that a mother could feel. She adored him and protected him as a child yet she deeply respected him as the man he had so abruptly become.

"I'm okay, mom. I'm not sick. I didn't sleep very well last night. It's another hectic finals week," he barely picked at his breakfast. "Sorry you went to all the trouble to make pancakes for me, but I'm not too hungry this morning," he apologized.

At the university that day his mind was blank. He shifted to automatic drive and answered all the questions on the anthropology exam without even reading them. He left the room with the sinking feeling of failure. At this point it didn't matter anyway.

It was 4:30 when he parked in front of Beth's house on Olive Street. She would be there alone because it was Friday. Her mother worked in the drugstore until 9:00pm on Fridays. He knocked softly. Beth, who had watched him get out of his car and walk up to the porch, opened the door instantly. He stood before her, the picture of dejection. She had never seen this side of him before. She felt pangs of remorse and foreboding.

She took his hand and led him to the couch, that soft retreat where they had held each other so many times. This is where they had escaped from reality and now this is where they would have to face it head on.

Malcolm broke the uncomfortable silence, "I would be lying to you if I said I'm happy about this. The timing is disastrous. If I was looking for an excuse to avoid the grueling next few years of medical school, I sure would have an out. I've thought this through carefully and......" He was choking up now and hesitated in mid-sentence.

"Malcolm, I'm so sorry. It's all my fault," Beth was crying now.

He held her in his arms. She was sobbing on his shoulder.

He tried to calm her, "It's our fault, not your fault. You have our baby inside your body. That baby is part of me, too."

Beth relaxed slightly, her sobs lessening somewhat.

"This is a blessed event. This child was meant to be. We will both cherish it forever," he knew that he did not love Beth, but he knew that he would love their child without reservation.

"But how can we afford to have a baby right now? I won't be able to work much longer....I'm so sick all the time."

"Beth, you've heard me say many times that if a problem can be solved with money, it's not much of a problem. Here's my chance to prove that statement. It won't be easy. We'll learn the true meaning of *austere*, but first things first......will you marry me?"

"I've been married to you for a long time now. You have to ask that?" Beth was quick to reply, matter of fact.

"We have to make it legal, for the baby's sake. We need a certificate. I don't think we can involve your mother or my folks in this. We have to make a trip to Portland and look for a place to live on the hill by the med school. We'll go on across the Columbia to Vancouver and get married. It's a quick deal there....the laws are different. We'll go as soon as finals are over here," Malcolm's sense of urgency made it clear that his plan of action was predicated on expediency and budget.

This was the only way he understood how to solve a problem. He was deliberate and practical, as always. Beth was meek and unsure of everything. His strength amazed and propelled her forward. This set the tone for their life together.

Their Portland trip went exactly as planned, fast and frugal. On the drive up, they were naïve and hopeful. On the drive back, they were married and ready to weather the stormy road just ahead.

Malcolm had decided to be a medical doctor, in spite of the impossible odds.

Chapter VI

Mission Accomplished

The freshman year of medical school made his pre-med studies in Eugene look like kindergarten by comparison. He was more than challenged. He felt like a hole had been drilled into his head and a funnel inserted. The volume of new information filled the funnel to his brain to the brim. No matter how hard he tried to assimilate, he was always one step behind. Rote memory had always come naturally and easily to him, but this was overwhelming.

He had little time, money or energy left over for family life. Beth was very pregnant and alone much of the time. She did manage to cook dinner every evening despite the constant morning sickness that plagued her. They discussed their daily activities over a meager menu, because of Beth he took the time to eat regularly. The one hour a day, the dinner hour, he set aside to give her his undivided attention was enough for her. She knew it was a major sacrifice on his part and she was grateful for his effort. She never complained, was always supportive and catered to his every whim. His determination left her no choice.

A son, James, was born the following spring. Malcolm's paternal instincts bubbled over on his arrival. He was proud and pleased to take his turn at changing diapers and rocking James to sleep. Holding his son to his chest made him complete. He would always feel a special closeness to his first born.

For some unknown reason, that Malcolm did not have time to ponder, Beth's diaphragm was dysfunctional and a second child was born two years later. Malcolm loved this daughter with the same fervor he had his first born. He felt like a rich man even though his pockets were always empty. He worked two part-time jobs his junior and senior years to make ends meet. This meant he was home even less than the first two years, but Beth was totally satisfied to live in her small world of children. She was, in fact, one of them. As they matured even they left her behind.

Chapter VII

The Internship

Malcolm graduated from medical school in 1953. He insisted on interning at a county hospital because the learning experience was much greater with more patient care responsibility. Most graduates preferred a private hospital where the pay was better and the work much less demanding. One could earn as much as $300.00 a month there.

He was one of 33 interns at Harbor View County Hospital in Seattle. He earned $85.00 a month with free meals and laundry. His schedule was three days and two nights on duty, with every third night off. He could not support his family on those wages, so he borrowed $50.00 a month from his parents. This was the first money he had ever accepted from them throughout his college career, but he loved medicine and he would have traded any hardship for more knowledge and experience.

At Harbor View the interns were expected to dedicate one month to each service in a rotating fashion. His fourth service was neurosurgery. It was the greatest challenge of all.

"Welcome on board, Dr. McKenna," he was greeted by Dr. Walton, the first year resident. "This is Dr. Morris, the second year resident, and Dr. Plant, chief resident,"

Dr. Walton continued, reverently.

Dr. Plant was aloof and bored with these preliminaries. Dr. McKenna hated prima donnas, so he had an immediate dislike for the chief resident. The more he got to know Dr. Plant, the more convinced he was that his initial impression was correct.

The intern cared for the 22 patients on the service and went on daily rounds with the residents. His chart notes were carefully scrutinized and commented upon. Dr. Plant seemed never to find anything commendable about Dr. McKenna's observations. His attitude was always demeaning. He gave the impression he was wasting his time on these rounds, or so it seemed.

They stood around Mr. Jordan's bed one Monday morning.

"What's this progress report you wrote yesterday mean, McKenna?" he glared in Dr. McKenna's direction. "You think he has a subdural hematoma? Where's the evidence? He's been here for over three weeks now and no change. Look at these patellar reflexes," he gloated as he thumped the patient's knees in rapid succession. "Normal," he flashed his penlight into the patient's eyes hurriedly. "See, the pupils are RRE and react to L&A. Hand me your ophthalmoscope," he ordered. "Now look at that. The VP's are bounding. Here McKenna, you take a look, this is a good time for you to see a normal retina and optic disc."

"I did a complete neurological yesterday including the eye exam," McKenna was near to impertinent as he stood his ground.

"Then why are you saying he has a sub-dural?" Dr. Plant's patience seemed to be wearing a little thin as he directed a wilting look in McKenna's direction.

"I looked back over his admission history and physical. I even did a spinal tap yesterday. I have been following him daily for the ten days that I have been on this service. His mind is not the same. He talks different. He has different symptoms."

"So you did a tap, huh? You young interns amaze me. He had a tap in the beginning but I can't fault you for wanting to practice," he said condescendingly, "How did it go?"

Before Dr. McKenna could answer, Dr. Plant continued. "I know you got fresh red cells, everyone does in the beginning," Dr. Plant was trying hard not to be overly critical, but not too hard.

McKenna did not wilt but continued to present his case in spite of Plant's disinterest in his findings. The other residents were amused by such impertinence.

"He has a few fresh red cells in the xanthochromic fluid. I interpreted this to bear witness to a fresh bleed over the old one."

"McKenna, I told you before you spoke, that a bloody tap is usual for fresh interns. That's all you proved to me. You did a poor procedure. Don't feel bad. We all did in the beginning. We'll spend some time before you leave and I'll give you some pointers on a proper spinal tap."

"I had some practice last month on contagious diseases. I even diagnosed a severe pneumococcic meningitis in a comatose admission."

Plant interrupted, "McKenna, you amaze me. Your Graham stain technique was flawed, pneumococcic meningitis is rare. I'll wager it was Graham negative. In any case, a few spinal taps does not qualify you as expert."

He saw that it was futile to present his findings to the closed-minded Plant so he swallowed hard and remained silent.

"Let's move on to the next patient. We've wasted enough time on this alcoholic, homeless derelict that was brought in unconscious after a brawl. McKenna, I'm sure you must now recognize your naiveté in patient care. Next time direct your efforts to a more worthy cause."

McKenna treated that patient with high doses of IV Penicillin only. He knew that his Graham stain was therefore not negative. McKenna thought over this experience with Dr. Plant. He thought again about the wisdom of a county internship over a private one. He would never have been able to diagnose, do the lab, and treat a patient so specifically

in the private setting.

He carried away the axiom to always listen. Listen to the other doctors, listen to relatives and above all listen to the patient. The patient is handing you the diagnosis if you interpret and listen. He did not let the chief resident's tirade dissuade him from sitting at Jordan's bedside and listening to his gibberish. It was different gibberish now than it had been a week ago when they first met.

"Do you have pain?"

"No, but my head feels different."

"Different how?"

"I hear strange sounds."

"What kind of sounds?"

"Like water running in my head."

"Where? Point to it."

"Here," he pointed to his left ear.

McKenna visualized a walled-off left frontal cyst filled with blood that would flow when the head turned. The hematoma had to be frontal since all the reflexes were normal and left-sided and the sound was heard best with the left ear. He felt certain of the diagnosis but how would he ever convince Dr. Plant?

As it turned out he didn't have to talk again about this case to the chief resident. Grande rounds took place two days later. Dr. Robinson, a practicing neurosurgeon from Seattle, stood at the head of the circle around Jordan's bed. Next to him was the chief resident, Dr. Plant, and then the second and first year residents, in that order. The lowly intern was last in line at the foot of the bed.

Dr. Robinson thumbed through the chart for what seemed to be an eternity. The silence was deafening. McKenna enjoyed seeing the residents standing there uncomfortable, speechless and humbled. The attending physician exuded an air of confident control.

At last he spoke, "This patient has been vegetating here since rounds two weeks ago. He's bed-ridden and sullen. Does he ever speak?" He glanced at the chart again. "The last chart note here is interesting. Who's McKenna?"

* * *

All eyes turned to the foot of the bed. The residents seemed in a state of shock. Dr. Robinson had by-passed the chain of command and was speaking to the intern.

"McKenna, I see you think this man has a subdural. How would you think this is possible after all this time has passed? His neurological exam is normal by your own admission."

The chief resident started to speak but was cut short.

"I'm asking Dr. McKenna," the attending blurted, almost rudely.

McKenna was startled and speechless for a moment. Finally he mustered up enough courage to reply, "Sir, this man's speech and mental acuity has changed since I first saw him two weeks ago. That fact and the normal neurological findings suggest it has to be a frontal hematoma."

"Has to be? What makes you think all these doctors here would miss something as obvious as a subdural? Even I didn't buy that when I saw him shortly after admission."

Not wanting to offend this surgeon who had practiced for more than twenty years, Dr. McKenna suddenly realized what thin ice he was skating on. "I do not want to come across as impertinent, sir. You are the expert here. I really……….."

Dr. Robinson cut him off. "Nurse, get this man ready for twist drill holes. Dr. McKenna wants to prove his point."

The residents smiled and McKenna cringed. *What have I gotten myself into*, he asked himself. No one spoke until the sterile bedside tray was set up.

"McKenna, those gloves are for you," Robinson broke the long silence.

"But I have never......"

"I'll walk you through. It's a simple procedure. You're here to learn, right?"

McKenna hoped no one would notice his hands shaking as he donned the sterile gloves.

They didn't. He appeared confident, as he always did, not wanting anyone to see his inner fear.

"Now fill the syringe with the Novocain. Where are you going to go in with the first hole?"

McKenna betadined the left frontal region and placed the hole in the drape there, "Like I said, sir, it will be here."

Dr. Robinson smiled, "So you did, so you did. Now that you have injected the scalp, make a half inch incision down to the skull. That's fine. Compress the area until we get the drill ready. Look at that drill carefully, you can see that it is designed to stop when you reach the dura. It's really not a big deal. People seem to think the skull is somehow sacred. It's not. We have to go through it to see the brain. It's that simple." He was skillfully guiding McKenna's every move.

Beads of moisture were coming out on McKenna's forehead. His gloves were damp inside. He poised the drill over the fresh incision. "Now remember, the drill will stop when you reach the dura," encouraged Robinson. The whirring sound of the drill added to the drama of the scene. A man's skull was about to be invaded, as if a carpenter and not a doctor was at work here. McKenna was in awe at what he was doing for the first time. He was almost surprised to see the dura so soon. It glistened at the bottom of the hole, looking thick and impenetrable.

"That's fine....now wipe the bone dust out and use the largest needle there."

McKenna picked up the heavy duty instrument that seemed too rigid to be called a needle. It pierced the dura with an ominous ease.

"Now remove the stylus," Robinson's voice was friendly and hopeful.

Black oil spurted from the needle.

Robinson turned to the nurse, "Schedule this man for surgery tomorrow morning. McKenna will be my assistant."

That pronouncement was electric. The resident's smiles had changed from amusement to amazement. McKenna was too stunned to enjoy his victory. He could not imagine that his future in medicine was sealed by this single event. His pure analytical mind would heal the sick and many times confuse and confound those who envied him.

Chapter VIII

Out of the Academic Cradle

Word travels quickly in a small county hospital community. Dr. McKenna was so busy completing his internship that he gave little notice to the respect he now received from the other residents. He admitted and cared for each new patient with such enthusiasm and brilliance that they would have had to dig very deep to find fault in any event.

A third child was born to the McKennas at Harbor View. The pressure was on Malcolm to start private practice for financial reasons. He was so eager to be a family doctor that this was secondary to him. He gave little thought to the fact that they drove a 1936 Chevrolet that burned more oil than gasoline or that there was no money for movies or meals out. He had no time for such foolishness. Beth was a Stepford wife and happy with her brood and that she had never had to work outside the home because of them.

Malcolm logically concluded that he would have to go into a salaried practice with an established clinic. Two such opportunities were available in the spring of 1954, a few months before his graduation. One was in the small town of Cashmere, in eastern Washington, the other in another small town, Stirling, east of Portland, Oregon. He really wanted to settle down in Eugene, Oregon, where he was born, but such an opportunity didn't present itself.

Dr. Ross, in Cashmere, was drawn to the fresh eagerness of McKenna. He was tired and needed help badly. Dr. McKenna liked Dr. Ross but somehow felt uncomfortable in Cashmere, the home of Aplets and Cotlets. He wanted to return to Oregon, the place that felt like home to him. Dr. Welch of Stirling was less personable than Ross, but he obviously was under pressure and felt the burnout that a small town doctor faces after a few years. Dr. McKenna saw an opportunity in Stirling to prove himself while making a good income to supply his growing family with their necessities. He could have gone on to specialize were it not for that fact. He gave that little thought because he really liked people and family practice suited him.

Dr. Alex Welch was reluctant to offer a salary as enticement because he had hired a young doctor recently who had not worked out and it cost him money, money that he could ill afford to pay because he was, as most doctors are, a poor office manager. He had an increasing flow of patients and overhead but a lagging cash flow. He could see, however, that McKenna was eager, so eager that he accepted the $500.00 a month salary without complaint. To McKenna, $500.00 was a huge increase over his $85.00 intern salary and he hoped to learn from this busy established MD.

"I have no way of knowing what you can do and I've been taken advantage of recently," Alex complained during their initial interview.

"I won't disappoint you," Malcolm reassured, ignoring the red flags that Welch raised whenever he spoke.

"We'll start out with $500.00 a month the first year and then see how it goes."

"Fine with me," money was never on Malcolm's mind. Treating patients was, and he saw a lot of those in the waiting room.

"Ed Moore, a patient of mine, has a house near here that he will rent you for $85.00 a month."

"Tell him I'll take it."

It was late June, 1954 when Malcolm backed a trailer he found in the want-ads up to the door of their unit. All they owned was a refrigerator and a rocking chair that was purchased with most of the $550.00 he got from the sale of his old army jeep during the first year of medical school. They also loaded some bunk beds and a kitchen table that had been acquired from an outgoing intern the year before. They padded these items with blankets and old clothes. Tied down with a canvas tarp to hide their meager load and protect it from the rain, the old Chevrolet gallantly pulled that load and the large family inside with only two rest stops. Each time the five gallon can of oil in the trunk rejuvenated the thirsty engine. It was on the Interstate Bridge, between Washington and Oregon, when a minor tragedy struck. The tarp somehow freed itself of the rope tie-down and was flapping in the wind like a giant sail. McKenna, for an instant, felt the pangs of poverty when he viewed the spectacle behind with its pathetic contents.

"The good news is, we didn't lose anything," he proudly proclaimed as he retied the rope.

The kids were laughing and Beth was stoic, as usual, at the adventure of it all. Inside, however, Malcolm felt the burden of the scene he had just been witness to. That thought was quickly dispersed by the optimism of what lay ahead.

"We are in Oregon now, our new home. Wait 'til you see the big house we'll have."

Beth was navigator in the front seat. "It looks like Burnside Street angles southeast to Stirling......that's the most direct route.......see?" She held the map to show him.

Malcolm was in no way familiar with east county though they had lived in west Portland, where he attended University of Oregon Medical School. Unfortunately, Burnside Street dead-ended in Rockwood before they reached Stirling. He backed up the trailer, with much difficulty, to turn around.

"Don't laugh, kids. I can do it! Remember, now, I never want to hear any of you say *can't*. Wipe it out of your vocabulary right now. Okay?"

They arrived at their new home on Third Street at 4:00 p.m. It was a surprise because none of them, including Malcolm, had seen it before.

Beth was first to speak, "It looks like a mansion compared to that Seattle condo."

She never complained while they lived there, in fact, she never complained about any of the hardships they had endured. This was part of her agreeable style. Malcolm, at times, felt guilty that he had been such a poor provider for his growing family. That was about to change.

Chapter IX

A New Doctor in Town

His first day at the office was a disappointment when only two new patients were sent his way. He heard the endless parade of footsteps outside his office door being ushered into Dr. Welch's rooms. He now realized how diluted challenging cases would be in private practice when he treated Tommy Bartlet's ear infection and Melody Trainer's wrist sprain.

He felt even more humbled as he walked to his 1952 well-used Plymouth in the parking lot. He thought a successful doctor should be seen in something like Welch's new 1955 Chrysler. He sobered to the realization that the $50.00 payment was even more than he could afford now. He didn't dwell on material problems like this for long.

"When I'm as busy as Welch, that money problem will take care of itself," he thought reassuringly.

He really hated to be bothered with the earthy problems of everyday life. He wanted to cure the sick, to be so busy that there was no time for the mundane.

He didn't have long to wait for his wish to become reality. Within three months his appointment calendar was full. Small town gossip centered on the young, handsome doctor.

"He's very young, and fresh out of training, but he's so interested in my problems…I really like him," Melody told her friends.

Like wildfire the word spread and Dr. McKenna found he was literally swamped and extremely happy and satisfied. Within six months he was busier than the well established Dr. Welch. This was a harbinger of the problems to come.

During the first few weeks, when he had time on his hands, he kept his eye on the office collections or actually the lack thereof. When he discovered that Dr. Welch, as busy as he was, was only taking home about twice his own meager salary he was perplexed. He was no economics major but did excel in math, so it was easy for him to deduce that an overhead figure of 80-90% was unrealistic. A big part of the problem was a low collection rate of 50%. In other words, half the patients were not paying or at best, paying very little. Why?

Dr. Welch never bothered to question such things. He left it up to the bookkeeper. She was an efficient and agreeable lady who had no reason to question anything, as long as the money was there for payroll. Dr. McKenna, on the other hand, felt he should receive reasonable payment for his services. He needed the money badly. He knew he was being paid less than the carpenter and plumber patients he saw, and a fraction of the salary the local business men were paid.

He presented his case to Dr. Welch after business hours one evening. Alex Welch was writing on charts and in a hurry to get home. He listened with polite disinterest.

"You have my permission to check all this out, McKenna. I'm too busy right now, as you can see. If you uncover anything worthwhile, let me know. I have dinner guests coming this evening, so I'll see you in the morning."

Malcolm was not disillusioned by his partner's brush off. On the contrary, he took it to mean he was free to manage the office. He filled that void efficiently, much to the chagrin of Maggie, the bookkeeper, who had been with Dr. Welch from the beginning when they had operated out of his home…just the two of them.

He instituted a rigid collection policy and raised the antiquated $3.00 office fee to $4.50. He knew that it cost them $1.50 to process an insurance claim. In a few months Dr. Welch's salary doubled and he felt obligated to tell Dr. McKenna that their agreement was voided and that they were now equal partners. His new associate had been there only six months and Dr. Welch was wise enough to value his worth and keep him happy to stay on. He wasn't wise enough, however, to see or admit that this young doctor was about to outdo him in every way. If he had been so observant and unpresuming, he could have avoided the heartaches they both would suffer much later. It had been foreseen that "such a pure analytical mind would heal the sick and confuse and confound those who envied him," and now it was coming to pass.

And heal the sick he did, hundreds of them, spreading the word. He was on a merry-go-round of his own making that he could not escape. He was indispensable. He was young. He was content in his little walled-off world where he was in complete control. His Stepford wife, Beth, fit nicely into that scheme of things too. She was happy with her growing brood of five and no financial restraints. She loved this amazing man and she thought he loved her. All was right with her world.

Malcolm viewed himself quite the contrary. He was a disease fighter. He made people well and reveled in their gratitude. He had self-doubts about those he couldn't help. He knew that medicine was not really the exact science that he wanted it to be. But he also knew that if he taxed his brain enough he could enjoy the cutting edge. He could do what was not expected. He could try harder and accomplish more.

Organized medicine, the politically correct group that controls medical societies, and in turn, all doctor's credentials, does not adhere to that philosophy. They prefer followers, not leaders. They are easily confused and prone to envy. The more successful Dr. McKenna became, the more he would be in their sights. He was not oblivious to them and would eventually have to deal with it.

A new doctor in town usually gets a few challenging patients that the old timers don't need or want. Maggie Black would certainly fall into that category. He was called one evening to make a house call.

"Maggie is being difficult again. We need your help. She refuses to go to bed," complained the exasperated caller.

"Does she have a regular doctor?"

"No, not really. She has been seen in the past, up at the county hospital, but they don't make house calls."

"I know. I'll be there within the hour," Malcolm wrote the address hurriedly on the pad by the telephone and was on his way within minutes.

Little did Dr. McKenna know how challenging this house call would be. He did know that a welfare case would be a write-off in terms of payment, but he was always anxious to help where he could. He felt confident he could handle anything. When he arrived, the woman who had called greeted him. It was Maggie's daughter, Frances.

"My mother is in her room over there. She's been in there for hours and won't come out."

About that time, the loud sound of breaking glass resounded throughout the house. They stepped into the doorway of Maggie's room just in time to see the sewing machine sailing through the air.

"Oh no, she just threw it out the window!" her daughter exclaimed in dismay.

Dr. McKenna tried to keep his composure noting that all the furniture in the small bedroom was in complete disarray.

"Does she have such violent spells often? Is she on any drugs?" he inquired.

"No, this is the first time for this. She does become despondent at times and she won't take pills."

Dr. McKenna was at a total loss for a plan of action but when Maggie sat down on the edge of her bed, he knew this was the time to establish a rapport with the patient. He walked over, sat down beside her, and placed his bag on the floor in front of him. He felt a friendly gesture should precede giving her an injection of a sedative.

"Maggie, I'm Dr. McKenna. I've come to help you."

Maggie stared into space.

"I will give you an injection that will make you feel peaceful. You will enjoy that feeling."

Maggie stared into space.

"I'll open my bag now to get the medicine," he said in a gentle soothing voice, all the while watching her out of the corner of his eye.

Maggie suddenly erupted into action, kicking his bag across the room. Bottles, tape and bandages were rolling in all directions. She turned and fell across him, all 250 pounds of her, pinning him to the bed. He was helpless. To add insult to injury, she grabbed his necktie. He was choking!

Frances and her stunned husband stood in the doorway, frozen into immobility. Dr. McKenna used every ounce of his strength to flip Maggie over and off him.

He held her down and ordered, "Call the sheriff's office and get someone over here, now. This is an emergency and I need you to help me hold her down until they get here."

After she was cuffed, he gathered up his equipment and gave her an injection.

As he drove away he laughed at himself, "It sure is hard to look professional with a 250 pound mad woman sitting on your chest and choking you with your own necktie!"

Another memorable house call occurred only a week later. The call came on Thursday at 2:15am. Dr. McKenna, who was physically battered from Wednesday's muscle stretching hobby-farming, did not move. After eight or ten abrasive rings, Beth nudged him gently, her left elbow cutting like a knife into the sonorous reverberations of his open-mouthed tortured dream. He pursed his lips against his arid, swollen tongue and attempted to speak, all while fighting a vision of looking down at himself staked spread-eagle in the desert sun, unable to move his aching arms and legs, his mouth parched from days of unquenched thirst.

At last his medical aplomb surfaced and he groped desperately for the phone to remove it before another ring would awaken his overly-protected wife. Still unable to articulate, he fought for orientation while an excited male voice on the other end of the line gradually achieved lucidity.

"Doc, it's coming…it's coming! You'd better get here real soon! Carrie is huffing and puffing like a donkey engine. She says it's coming and always before when she said it's coming, it came. Hurry up, Doc…hurry on over here, before all this hot water gets cold. She won't wait much longer, I tell you!"

At last the name *Carrie* penetrated his brain and he was suddenly completely aware that the frantic unanswered dialogue was that of Ralph Fedders, a patient he had seen several times in the office.

"Slow down now, Ralph," arumph, arummpphh, he cleared his throat, "you mean Carrie is in labor?" At last McKenna managed a croaking low-pitched voice.

"In labor,…hell, Doc…she's having her baby right here and now!"

"Okay….okay, Ralph…I'm on my way," he was now sitting on the edge of the bed as he hung up the phone.

He reached down to the floor in front of him and managed to come up with a pair of socks and some shorts. These he clutched protectively as he staggered slowly towards the bathroom.

There he muttered under his breath from the throne, "Why do all these damn babies have to come in the middle of the night?"

He pulled on his socks and then stepped into the shorts as he arose, now completely awake. He expertly and quietly found his clothes in the darkness of the bedroom so that Beth would not be disturbed. He was always very thoughtful when it came to his wife. As he was leaving he looked down at her motionless silhouette and said under his breath, not wanting to disturb her sleep, "Bye sweetheart, I'll be back soon."

But was she really asleep? Had he caught the phone quickly enough? His question was answered when he stealthily left the room and she called after him as she had a hundred times before.

"Drive carefully, darling, you know all the crazy people are out this time of the night."

Dr. McKenna's farm was only a mile from the Fedders. He arrived in ten minutes. He pulled into the driveway and could see that the back porch light was on. The front entry was blocked with old farm equipment and a huge pile of tires. He walked up the dilapidated, creaky back stairs. The hand rail was loose and unstable. Nestled between an old metal hot water heater and a rickety stepladder was the back door. It was open. He walked into a kitchen that smelled sour. Opened bottles and empty food containers were piled in disarray everywhere he looked.

"Where are you?" he called into the darkness.

"Back here, Doc. Follow the light to the bedroom."

He walked toward the faint glow at the end of the hall. His shoes seemed to stick to the floor. He hoped it was jelly and peanut butter. To his left he saw a couch where someone was sleeping, the soft hum of snoring filled the room. This must be the living room, he thought. He reached the lighted doorway and saw a very tired Carrie Fedders sitting up in bed proudly holding a fully dressed baby, a pink ribbon fastened in her hair. In a corner of the room four small children slept, all in a row, on a thick blanketed mattress. Ralph was sitting on the bed holding his wife's hand.

"Where is the afterbirth? I need to see it," he asked Ralph.

"I threw it out the back door, Doc. I'll get it."

While he was gone, McKenna examined the baby. He examined the placenta. It was intact, not surprisingly, since the mother was not bleeding and had no tears. The seven other births that had preceded this miracle had seen to that.

"Bring the baby into my office in six weeks....... or sooner if you have problems," he told them. He did not send a bill for no services rendered.

A few months into his practice, the chart he pulled from the holder on the door of room 3 was labeled baby Holmes, age three months. He entered and looked directly into the worried face of Mrs. Holmes. Her baby, Alice, was crying over her shoulder and facing away from him. Malcolm knew instantly that this was not just another baby with colic. The mother's look and the baby's incessant loud cry, with knees drawn up, was atypical.

"Hello, Mrs. Holmes, so we have a sick baby here."

"Yes, doctor, she's been crying since 3 a.m. She's worn out and won't nurse," her voice trembled with exhaustion, "I'm at my wit's end."

"Does she have abnormal BMs or dark urine?" he questioned as he took the baby and gently laid her on the exam table. "Has she had a cold?"

"No," the tired mother replied.

A baby cannot speak for itself and symptoms are always completely different than in an adult. Dr. McKenna's every move and demeanor was calm and reassuring. He was silent as he methodically probed the baby's abdomen with the flat of his hand and then with his index and middle fingers. He was watching the facial expressions and leg movements at the same time. He listened to the chest and abdomen with his stethoscope. He looked in her throat and ears. He noted the date on the chart was followed by a recorded normal rectal temperature and pulse rate. He turned the baby over and examined her back and neck. He thumped her right and left kidney area just below the rib cage. He did a rectal exam.

"Mrs. Holmes, we will need to admit your baby to Providence Hospital for some tests and I'll have a surgical consultant see her. She has something going on in her right lower abdomen. We must rule out appendicitis."

"I didn't know babies got that."

"It is rare and very difficult to diagnose. Let's see what develops. If it is, and found early, we can operate on babies with no more danger than an adult," he reassured her.

Dr. Carter, the surgical consult, agreed with the diagnosis of appendicitis and surgery was performed that afternoon. The procedure went well and lasted a little over one hour. Dr. Carter checked on the patient that evening and reassured the parents that all was well.

"She's doing better than expected at this point and will likely be discharged in three or four days. I'd advise you to hang onto that Dr.McKenna, he made a prompt, very difficult diagnosis."

They did. Alice had grown into a beautiful, young woman of 22 when she and her new husband moved away from Stirling.

The range of family practice was portrayed at the other end of the age scale by Miss Mina Mondale. Miss Mondale, a retired old-maid school teacher, was 84 years of age when he saw her early one rainy March day, the second year of his practice. He liked her instantly. Her tiny feet and the great big smile that never left her face, were the first things he noticed about her. She was such a delightful human being, her cheerfulness was contagious and ever present. That feeling was mutual because he was her doctor until her death at 107.

"Do you remember that first visit I made to your office?" she asked him with a chuckle fifteen years after the fact.

"No, Mina, I've always prided myself on a good memory but it's nothing like yours. You even remember the birthdates of all my kids and ask about them by name which is amazing to me. What about that first visit?"

"Well, I was sitting in the corner, across from the door, when you opened it and I said to myself, 'Can that young whippersnapper really know enough to take care of me?'" she laughed louder now and added, "You have kept me well all these years and I must say thank you so much."

"That's okay, Mina, I should thank you for the legion of patients you have sent to me."

"They all love you too, Dr. McKenna, what would we do without you?"

She was the guest of honor at his home at a party to celebrate her 100th birthday. She had no car and her little size two shoes were still carrying her into the office.

Chapter X

Those Other Women

Mina was by far the oldest, but not his only, female admirer. Rumors were rampant about the handsome, young doctor. According to some, the hospital nurses, his office nurses, most attractive patients and many others yet to be identified were all conquests of Dr. McKenna. The trail of envy continued.

He did admire all things of beauty, that was a given. As an ardent fly fisherman he felt refreshed by the great outdoors. He thought the snow-covered peaks of the Cascades were put there by God's hand to humble man. He felt the same about women. He admired them from afar but under his circumstances, felt honor bound to view them as he did the distant mountain peaks. Lascivious thoughts with female patients never crossed his mind. His passion for healing and need to cure ailments crowded out and replaced all else.

When an occasional patient became flirtatious, he always laughed and tried to diffuse the situation with a joke. He had a way about him that was disarming, even in the most uncomfortable moments.

Mrs. Crown presented him with a new and far more challenging problem than he had ever been confronted with before. She had been a devoted patient for several years and at no time did she give so much as a hint at being seductive. She didn't appear to be the type, a fifty-one year old, happily married woman, with grown children. The empty nest syndrome may have precipitated the anxiety for which he was treating her. It was late afternoon, on a Wednesday, when a call came in from her. She said she had fallen and hurt her back and neck and didn't want to move until he saw her. He made a house call on his way home at 5:30.

Her driveway was parallel to another, which led to an adjoining garage, so that her front porch was only about thirty feet from the front door of the neighbor. He drove in and parked in front of her garage. He walked to her door, bag in hand. This black case was given to him when he graduated from medical school by a family friend, Hazel. She had been a nurse in Pennsylvania with his Aunt Ted. They migrated to Oregon together in the late twenties. The bag was very large and bi-folded so that two departmental shelves held every manner of drugs, needles and instruments. He treated every kind of illness from this well used, monogrammed pharmacy.

He pressed the door bell button and was shocked to see Melanie Crown open the door. He had expected her to be lying on the floor with her daughter comforting her. His amazement was deepened by the fact that she was dressed, or you might say undressed, in a filmy negligee.

"Come in, doctor."

He found himself stepping into a well rehearsed, well laid out romance novel of her making.

"I know you will want to examine my back," she purred and headed directly to her bedroom.

He was living page 26 of her novel when his eyes followed her long shapely bare legs. Her flowing dark hair extended half way down that suntanned expanse of skin that finally gave way to a perfectly rounded gluteus maximus. A stunned silence betrayed his surprise.

She moved onto the bed with a seductive ease that an injured back would not have allowed. Posed with one leg extended and the other angled to present an inviting thigh, she breathed deeply to say, "I have wanted you for years and now I have you…..come over here and examine me."

Malcolm, for once in his life, was speechless. This tempting vision, so available, had to be unreal. He pulled himself up from the spell she was casting, to gather his thoughts. Professionalism must always trump temptation. The words leaped to the forefront of his mind and stayed there. But he was at a loss as to how to deal with this situation.

She sensed his confusion and spoke with determination, "If you don't get in this bed now I will scream for help and let me caution you the neighbors are home."

At that moment the repercussions hit him in the gut. He visualized the headline in the local paper, DOCTOR RAPES PATIENT. No one would believe that he was the victim.

He sat on the edge of her bed and took her extended hand.

He looked into her eyes and spoke with a sincerity born of desperation, "Melanie, you are a beautiful, desirable woman and I would be lying if I said I wasn't flattered…….. But we are both married. We have children. It is not possible for this to happen."

He sat with her in silence feeling bad for her and wishing he could say something more that would ease the suffering that had brought her to such a confrontation.

Tears flooded her cheeks as she spoke, "Of course you are right. You are always right. It's just that I do love you."

He wiped her tears away as he answered, "You are such a fine woman. Your husband is a very lucky man. I will always be there for you."

He picked up his bag and as he was leaving the room he turned to say, "This never happened."

Beth was an eager participant in his adrenalin charged performance that night. She was blessed with an uninhibited sexuality and always available. It was undoubtedly because of this that he overlooked all of her shortcomings. They never argued.

Much later, in his practice, another Melanie Crown incident almost happened, except this time the gorgeous Hilary was more spontaneous. She did not think through her plan carefully. It was about 10 pm when her phone call came. Malcolm was propped up in bed reading a medical journal.

"This is Hilary Smith….I need you to come over now."

"What's your problem?" He was perplexed because Hilary had never called after hours before and she sounded more agitated than ill.

"I need to talk to you now," she emphasized the *now*. She was flustered and hesitant.

"How about if we talk in the office tomorrow, it's pretty late," the tired Malcolm suggested.

"Oh…Alright then," she hung up.

She did not report to the office the next day so Dr. McKenna thought he must have been correct in assuming the pampered Hilary was just looking for more attention. Had she cleverly invented an illness as Melanie Crown had done, he would have made that house call.

It was about two weeks later when he saw Dr. Weinstein, the Mt. Hood College president, who was a long standing patient.

"Oh my God, Doc, it must be true, all those rumors about women!" Earl was laughing boisterously, as he was prone to do.

"What do you mean?"

"You haven't heard about Hilary Smith then?" Earl was always tuned into the college scuttlebutt where Hilary's husband, James, was a professor.

"She caught her husband with another woman and she just went berserk!" Earl felt he could share secrets with his doctor and they would remain with him. "I heard she was a virgin when they married which made things worse."

He had expected some sort of reaction from McKenna but none was forth coming so he continued, "She threatened that she would have an affair to even the score."

A long pause ensued.

"I think that's where you come in, Doc."

"That's interesting, Earl, but what does that have to do with me?"

"Her husband laughed at her and asked her, "Who with?" and she said 'With Dr. McKenna, naturally,'" Earl laughed again. "You're one lucky s.o.b., she's a doll."

"Wait a minute. I've had no affair with Hilary," Dr. McKenna now knew what that phone call had been all about.

He had dodged yet another bullet.

Dr. Weinstein left the office that day wondering if his doctor was human. He wanted all the rumors to be true because for the last year or so he had harbored an unbearable desire to have an affair with Jill, the doctor's new trophy wife. He, too, was a high profile professional in this small town and Jill knew nothing about his feelings which hampered his plans.

Chapter XI

Beth and Malcolm

In college, when Malcolm began to feel a serious attraction to women, there was Beth. She was petite, blonde, quiet and sultry. Her kisses were remarkable. If there had been such a thing as a kissing competition she would have taken first place and gone on to win the nationals.

She set her sights on the studious junior class president. His limited experience and her innate warmth were a perfect fit. She taught him to enjoy the instinctive side of life that he had failed to find in the books he loved so much. They were married when he entered medical school, three years later.

Beth became a Stepford wife. She was stoic and never complained about the financial hardships they would have to endure. They found a one room, $35.00 a month rental, a few blocks from the medical school. The small house faced east and the wintry blast from the Columbia Gorge hit the hilltop with a penetrating coldness. The bay window, where Malcolm placed his study desk, absorbed that frigidity like a sponge wicking up moisture. He wrapped his feet with a blanket on windy days to keep the chill away. The only sink was in the tiny bathroom. Their kitchen consisted of a row of wooden orange crates with a piece of plywood across the top to create much needed counter space. Oil cloth hung over the front opening allowing the crate's middle partition to act as shelving for plates and pans. A two-burner hot plate on the counter top served as an electric range. Water was carried from the bathroom sink and heated there. Malcolm had to sell his prized Army jeep to buy a much-needed refrigerator and rocking chair. The remainder of the furniture, including their bed, was hand-me-downs. He preferred to call them family heirlooms. The cradle for their first-born, a hooded wicker antique, truly was a treasure. It had surely been used with loving tenderness for many years before the McKennas were lucky enough to find it one spring day at the Eugene flea market. In spite of the constant chill in the air, James grew up to be healthy and always warm-blooded.

Pregnancy forced Beth to quit her job which would have helped so much at this time. Malcolm came very close to quitting on more than one occasion because of the intense pressure this double life created. His marriage to Beth was both his salvation and his nemesis. One night he did not return directly home after a study session at the library. He went there on a regular basis, because there was not enough money to buy many of the books he needed. He stopped at the market, near the school, and bought a bottle of cheap wine. He drove to the parking lot overlooking the twinkling city lights of Portland after dark. He stared out across the vast expanse of lights and real world.

He was not a drinker so that a few gulps of wine put his mind into a whirling escape. He thought about all those people below who were living normal lives, with normal jobs, and living in normal houses. They had no money worries. They were the smart ones. He was living an impossible double life; a father and husband and a nerdy student of medicine. How could he do a good job of either? He was floundering in this rough sea of life and sharks were everywhere. He dozed off. His mental fatigue and the wine didn't mix well or perhaps they did, because he awoke an hour later, refreshed, and drove home eagerly. Beth greeted him at the door.

"Where have you been? I've been worried," she enveloped him in her warm embrace and kissed him passionately.

She did not wait for an answer but took him into the bedroom and undressed him. Her body was much better than wine.

Beth did not change, but he did. As his practice flourished, healing the sick so successfully was heady stuff. Now he had another double life to deal with; the practice and his even larger family. Medicine has been called a jealous mistress and it was. He found himself drawn more and more into the whirlpool of his practice, for which he was so well suited.

Beth could feel him slipping away but was helpless. She just loved him and his children and hoped. She knew he was such a good man that however he coped she would be a partner to it without question.

It all started innocently enough. When he felt smothered by the small town where he was on the head of a pin, displayed like a butterfly, he would fly away to prove that he was not dead yet. He would travel to medical meetings in far away places like Las Vegas, LA and Mexico, where he was unknown and free. Beth stayed home and enjoyed the children. When he returned with his batteries recharged, she was at the door to welcome him. She never questioned what her Alexander did on his crusades.

His adventures always took unexpected turns and proved to be challenging to his creativity. On a side trip to Las Vegas, from LA, his unexpected companion was Marie Collier. She was a lead love interest on a TV series. He did not have much time for television but knew that this drop-dead gorgeous woman, who boarded United Flight 1140 in LA, must be a celebrity. He had walked to the front section of the sparsely booked 737 because he liked to sit where there was plenty of leg room. Seats all around him were vacant so he was surprised when Marie took the seat next to him. He had taken the window seat. She ignored him in haughty silence.

"What kind of game is this?" he thought, "Why sit so close in a nearly empty plane and then appear so disinterested?" He used his best bed-side manner conversation.

"My name is Malcolm McKenna."

She responded without looking from the magazine she was using as a prop, "Marie Collier."

"I've been to a meeting in LA and I'm heading to Vegas to make my fortune," he small talked. She said nothing so he continued, "You have Hollywood written on your forehead. My guess is you're escaping too."

"You've got that right."

Then uncomfortable silence again while she stared at the magazine.

He carried on a ten-minute dialogue about nothing important. He surprised himself at how humorous some of it was. He had exhausted all the small talk he could conjure up when she looked over toward him with a disarming smile.

"You are cracking me up....where did you come from?" The ice was broken and he found out that she could talk after all.

"I vowed that I would talk to no one on this trip. I'm burned out. I just want to be alone."

"I'll call you Garbo then, how about that? You can be incognito. I won't blow your cover if you'll do likewise. I'm trying to escape from burnout too. Not as glamorous as yours, but burnout nonetheless. I'm a butterfly on a pin framed for all to see. I am in suspended animation and cannot fly......well, not until this plane takes off anyway."

It was totally out of character for him to enjoy such meaningless chatter but he was really pumped and in awe of the mysterious beauty sitting so near.

"You're a butterfly? Well, I will admit, you do look harmless enough and I mean that in the nicest way. Are you harmless?"

"Not really," he smiled his best disarming smile. "But I could lose my head and go berserk around a beauty like you. God knows what I would do."

"Somehow I'm completely at ease with you. I'm not with most men. Why is that? What do you really do when you're not on the pin?"

"I heal the sick. I'm a small town M.D. from Oregon, no less."

"That explains it," she said, visibly relaxing. "I've always admired doctors. It must be that dedication thing that puts me at ease. They exude trust but you also exude pheromones," she laughed, "I like that combination. Don't be too defensive about the small town thing. I'm from Fargo, North Dakota."

"We do have a lot in common, you and me. I would like to know what makes you tick though. Your beauty is way too distracting," he was serious now and she sensed that shift.

"How would you like to spend this evening with me? I could show you the real, behind- the-scenes, Vegas. I was a dancer there before I went to Hollywood."

"You're on."

This latest adventure was unfolding rapidly and very much to his liking.

Vegas was small and intimate in those days and he was proud to be escorting the most beautiful girl there that night. They danced and talked the night away. She introduced him to every casino manager and to a bevy of entertainment beauties. None were her equal, however. She was in a class by herself.

Time was on a different schedule that night. It was revved up, just as they were, and it was 4:30 a.m. when they sat in the restaurant at the Sands for breakfast. They were famished. All of his energy was abruptly drained and he was suddenly aware that this woman was like the Mona Lisa, like the snow-covered mountain peaks back home. She was meant to be viewed from afar but not touched. She was all about herself. She had nothing to give. She was a shell, empty inside. Now he had to conjure up a way to politely exit the scene.

"Marie, I really had a good time. It was a blast seeing this town from the inside.....thanks. I know you had meant to have a low key rest and look what I did to that plan."

"Malcolm, the pleasure was all mine and I mean that sincerely. I really enjoyed your company. You are such a refreshing change from Hollywood. I feel as if I'm on a pedestal there. You're so real, so warm…a rarity in my life."

"I'm really sorry I have such an early flight home," he lied. Since they had met in the lobby after their flight, he didn't know if she was staying there or at another hotel. "Can I walk you to your place?"

"No, I'm staying with a girlfriend at her apartment. She will meet me here later."

They embraced and kissed for the first time. He had never kissed a Mona Lisa before. Her lips were cold, like his mountains back home.

"Goodbye….I'll look you up the next time I get to LA."

She had slipped her phone number into his pocket earlier. She looked so alone when he turned to wave.

"I've found such beauty and such warmth but always in different women," he mused as he fell asleep. "God help me if I ever find it all rolled into one."

He returned to Oregon and she returned to Hollywood. They would never meet again, but he never forgot her.

LA was the setting for another R and R when his alma mater, U of O, played in the Rose Bowl. His team narrowly lost 10 to 7 playing against a powerful Ohio State team. As it turned out he escaped another calamity by a razor thin margin on that New Year's Day, 1958.

Beth and Malcolm met Bill and Anne Osbourne, a dazzling Los Angeles beauty and her tag-along husband, at the Sands Hotel in Las Vegas in late 1956. Malcolm was taking a break from his hectic medical meeting schedule by the gold-tiled hotel pool when he noticed the disparate brunette lying in the shade of a palm tree. She was fully engrossed in the dog-eared manuscript in her hand. She exuded an aura of urgency and restlessness. Malcolm glimpsed a flicker of desperation in her eyes. He wondered if there was anything he could do to help and so he struck up a conversation with her husband, Bill, who had just completed five laps in the Olympic-sized pool.

Bill introduced Malcolm to his wife and they sat in the sun as a threesome for most of the afternoon while Beth was resting in their room upstairs. Malcolm discovered that the manuscript which Anne had been so intently reading earlier was a script from her agent in Los Angeles. She explained that this was her last chance to make a name for herself. The past ten years she had devoted entirely to her husband and children and now her fleeting moment of opportunity was nearly over. Malcolm hoped she would find the success she was searching for.

Later that evening, Beth and Malcolm were at the bar enjoying a beer when Anne tapped him on the shoulder wanting to know if they would like to join she and Bill at their table. It became obvious that Anne was slightly intoxicated when she talked openly about her untimely marriage to Bill which had cast a negative shadow on her fledgling acting career. Now with three small children she was totally trapped and desperately unhappy. Bill was embarrassed by his wife's confession at the dinner table, but humored her good naturedly nonetheless. Anne invited their new friends to spend the remainder of the evening cruising Las Vegas Boulevard in the Osbournes' red convertible. The next morning Anne was waiting in the Sands lobby to make good on her offer to drive Beth and Malcolm to the airport.

* * *

Two years later, as Malcolm rummaged through his disheveled desk drawer in search of his favorite black pen, he found Bill Osbourne's long lost business card. He remembered that Las Vegas evening spent talking and laughing with the couple. It seemed like so long ago and he wondered what they were both doing now.

Malcolm already had a trip planned to LA to see his alma mater, Oregon, play in the Rose Bowl. The smaller Northwest schools seldom had this opportunity and he didn't want to miss it. He was coveting four tickets to this glorious event which he had hidden away in his office safe.

He was beginning to feel the burn-out effects of his intense, non-stop work ethic. He had the distinct sensation that he was single-handedly supporting and nurturing not only his wife and family, but the entire town of Stirling. He craved the solitude and anonymity of the big city. He did, however, have those three extra tickets to the Rose Bowl and wouldn't mind having company during the game and to welcome the New Year. He never again wanted to be alone to celebrate this holiday after his unforgettable experience on the Maginot Line in France. That near-death event had left an indelible scar, like a deep scratch on a record. When the needle hit that spot the static was intolerable. Every New Year's he needed to be supported somehow and then all the rest of the year he would be able to bear the load.

In late November he wrote a letter to Bill Osbourne in LA and asked if he and Anne would like to see the game with him. He received a quick reply of acceptance and an offer to stay with the couple as their houseguest. He felt a thrill of anticipation at the thought of getting to know Bill and Anne better. He had enjoyed their brief interlude in Las Vegas. He remembered the couple as the perfect counterbalance; Bill's down-to-earth simplicity evening out Anne's Hollywood flair. This spontaneous experience was exactly what he needed to center himself in preparation for the continuous pressure he felt to be the ideal problem-solver and provider for all around him.

Unfortunately, he was stricken with an attack of appendicitis just before Christmas. He was still in the hospital recovering from surgery on December 25th. He developed a urinary tract infection and fever of 105 degrees as a complication. He was determined, however, to make the flight to LA on December 29th. He shouted orders to the nurse for Macrodantin immediately. She was perplexed by such a sick patient, especially since he was a doctor and knew better, demanding specific treatment. But she humored him and asked his doctor to legitimize the request. His fever responded and he was discharged on December 28th.

Beth, too, was perplexed when he asked her to pack his bag and drive him to the airport the next day.

"You're so pale and weak. You can barely walk because of the pain in your side," she chided him. "You have to be kidding…"

"I'm not kidding, Beth. I refuse to miss that game," he was adamant.

Knowing it was futile to argue, Beth packed his bag.

"I'll get you to the airport," she added under her breath. "I hope your unbelievable stubbornness gets you the rest of the way."

She knew it would. It always had.

Bill was waiting for him at LAX.

"My God, Doc, what happened to you?" he blurted out upon seeing the pale, gaunt figure limping toward him.

"I had my appendix out a few days ago, but I'm fine now," was Malcolm's ready excuse.

"I can see you really do need some R and R. You can lay in the sun by our pool," he offered sympathetically. "The weather has been unusually warm. It was 80 degrees yesterday."

Bill helped Malcolm walk slowly to the car. He hoped the sun would put some color back into those grayish cheeks.

"That sounds like a winner, Bill. How is Anne getting along these days?" Malcolm's question was punctuated with a grimace. His pain was obvious.

"She's in better shape than you, Doc," Bill laughed trying to lessen the gravity of this unexpected situation. "You're telling me you got out of the hospital only yesterday and you're here today?!"

"That's about it….I had no choice. This trip was very important to me."

"We'll see if we can make it memorable, Doc. You're an amazing guy," he said shaking his head and trying to understand this crazy turn of events.

They arrived 45 minutes later at a stately home in Palos Verdes. Bill ushered Malcolm through the door where he was confronted by a stunning vision in red. Anne's dazzling smile welcomed him to her home. Her warmth reassured him that he was exactly where he should be at this moment. He straightened to his full height, suddenly feeling no pain.

"Hello, Anne. You are even more beautiful than I remembered," he reached to shake her hand.

Instead she pulled him to her in a warm embrace and said, "You look like you need a hug. What happened?"

"Actually, I'm in the pink now," he grinned weakly. "You should have seen me a few days ago. My appendix was feeling its oats, but it's out now."

"You poor thing," her voice oozed sympathy, "I'll follow the doctor's orders and make you better. Just you name it and I'll do it for you."

After Bill left for the office the next morning, Anne made it very clear that she had fallen for Malcolm at their first meeting in Las Vegas. She described to him the tartan tie and tan suede leather coat he had worn, every word of conversation that had passed between them, the minute details of the way he laughed and the nuances of speech patterns that were his alone. She confessed she had sensed his loneliness then and it was even more apparent to her now.

"I know you need me," she said with certainty, "as much as I need you."

"Wait a minute, Anne. You and I are both vulnerable right now. Let's try to keep this relationship platonic," he protested, knowing he was fighting a losing battle.

He knew the next few days would be exceptional. They were that… and more. He was not disappointed.

Twice more in the following months he returned to Anne's waiting arms. When she began talking of marriage, of both of them leaving their children, reality set in. Malcolm had five small children at home. He could never abandon them. He would not return to LA again…..ever.

These escapes were like an overflow steam valve for Dr. McKenna. They were few and far between, but essential to preserve the sanity he desperately clung to in order to preserve his high profile existence back in small-town Stirling.

Shortly after his final visit to LA, Dr. McKenna saw a new patient. Bill Wise was having severe left flank pain that he correctly diagnosed and treated as a kidney stone. This case was unusual (and ironic considering Malcolm's recent time spent in the big city mecca) in that Mr. Wise had just moved to Oregon from LA. He had been treated for several years at UCLA for kidney stones. They had operated for the last one and he had a fresh right flank scar to prove it.

UCLA is considered cutting edge medicine so Dr. McKenna was reluctant to believe that Bill's personality changes and his easy fatigue could be related to the obvious problem of recurring kidney stones. He always felt that if one diagnosis could cover all the symptoms then just to go with it. So he did. He suspected a parathyroid adenoma. He had never seen one, but they did exist. He cracked some books, which he seldom had to do. His attention centered on a statement about spinal fluid calcium. In some cases, but not all, it could be slightly elevated. He smiled before closing the book that night. He went to sleep reliving the spinal tap incident on neurosurgery during his internship. He had performed many since then and was never bashful about using that invasive technique, setting him apart from most family doctors.

There were no reliable blood tests at the time for the rare tumor, so he proceeded that week with the spinal tap. The calcium level was slightly elevated, confirming his diagnosis. He didn't hesitate. UCLA be damned. He called in a general surgical consultant. Ten days later they opened Bill Wises' neck to explore his thyroid gland.

The surgeon, Dr. Huntington, had grown to respect the young doctor's judgment and asked, "Which side should we look at first?"

"The left side," McKenna stuck his own neck out. But he knew he had felt a slight prominence on the left.

"There it is!" the two doctors exclaimed simultaneously.

A pea-sized discrete tumor was nestled behind the left lobe of the thyroid.

"What damage such a little thing can do," Dr. Huntington commented sagely.

"You're right. Bill here has, over the past six years, had a total of eight kidney stones with pain that approaches childbirth. He's been getting very tired and dull of late too."

That surgery had been so short and so simple to put an end to years of such suffering. The Wises were extremely grateful and added to Malcolm's roster even more patients. He would diagnose two more parathyroid adenoma cases in the years that followed. Most doctors never see one such case in a lifetime.

Rare to Malcolm meant *possible*. He was never deterred by percentages but he seldom failed to find what he suspected.

"Make a diagnosis then test to prove it, not the other way around," was his mantra.

He learned by experience to trust only his own eyes and ears. Intermediaries always distort the truth. It was this minutia and responsibility that was thrust on him in never ending and greater amounts that took its toll and he gradually changed inside.

He saw the world as a place where forces worked against mankind. Nature was beautiful and hostile. Everything was designed to unsettle mankind. He witnessed death on its own terms. It was, in many cases, welcome relief.

"I must keep myself healthy and my brain clear so that I can always be here for all these people who need me," he thought frequently.

This pressure affected his home life. He was gone much of the time. Holidays were never sacred. That infernal phone would ring in the middle of Thanksgiving dinner or when the kids were around the Christmas tree. Beth, as good as she was, did not seem to understand him anymore. He became distant even when he was there.

Chapter XII

The Silent Partner

Dr. Alex Welch was in many ways ideal for this energetic, altruistic, young associate but they were complete opposites. He sat like a gruff bear in his office. He always seemed aloof and uncaring. If he was amazed at Dr. McKenna whirling around him, it didn't show. He enjoyed his rising income and kept silent, but down inside envy was taking its toll.

They would hold brief meetings on occasion to discuss business problems. It was always Dr. McKenna who controlled such meetings because Dr. Welch didn't seem to know problems existed. After only two years McKenna wanted to build a new office. The one they were leasing was becoming more and more oppressive. They were bursting at the seams with all the new patients and the central heating system created a literally smelly problem. Hot water floor heat was not appropriate for a doctor's office. McKenna would cringe when he walked out each evening, realizing how fresh the air smelled. All those bodies and the lack of air-conditioning were oppressive to him. The surgery located at the western side suffered the full effect of the hot afternoon sun. Dr. McKenna, who was in that suite much more of the time than Dr. Welch, suffered most.

After several months of pleading with his recalcitrant partner, he said in desperation, "If you don't see how critical this problem is, I'll build it myself."

Dr. Welch, who feared the cost of such a venture and had a son in college to support, did not sleep well that night. He was on the horns of a dilemma. Now might be a good time to rid himself of this unbearably productive young upstart. He thought back on his lonely practice before. He thought about his pocketbook then and now.

The following morning he surprised Dr. McKenna. "Let's build that new office. It is stuffy in here."

That's all Malcolm had to hear. He threw himself into the project. It would become his sculpted masterpiece.

First he spent his afternoons off visiting several offices in the Portland area. He observed not only the architecture but the flow of patients and the efficiency, or mostly lack thereof, of the personnel. He was surprised at the low volume and high overhead of these offices. He lay awake nights, hearing and seeing office personnel and patients flowing like a concerto. He loved music even though he was tone deaf and couldn't sing a note.

His new office was a work of art and the flow was musical, just as he had imagined it. He now had the perfect instrument to heal the sick. None would be turned away.

At first his lavish new private office amazed and pleased Dr. Welch. As time went on, however, the sounds outside his closed door were deafening. What was music to Malcolm, grated on Alex's nerves. The overhead went down and his salary went up with those decibels. He found himself drinking a few extra cocktails at night. When people on the street of this small town told him how wonderful his new doctor associate was, his stomach tightened. This was his town. He had been here years before McKenna. The old timers were his cronies. The politics were his and the mayor lived next door to his house up in the west hills. *Snob-knob* it was called.

Malcolm was in his glory and it never entered his head that his partner was in such a black mood. He would be brought down to earth and enlightened by a new Burroughs accounting machine that he researched and bought for the business office. How could a single 4x4 foot inanimate object clear his head so quickly? It was the first one installed in a doctor's clinic and would, many years later, be the last one cranking out patient ledgers.

Each month, from that time on, a printout of each doctor's production would catch the eye of the alert Dr. McKenna. He was dumbfounded. He was Dr. Welch's bread and butter…

* * *

It was 2 a.m. and he was driving home alone from Emanuel Hospital in Portland, a distance of about fifty miles. He had delivered a baby. His head had not hit the pillow and he was booked in at the office for an 8 a.m. complete physical. He gripped the wheel and stared into the night trying hard not to nod off into a sleep that his body was telling him it needed.

He thought, "What am I… a complete fool?"

He did the quick math deducting the overhead, state and federal taxes. Then he divided the small balance by two. One half of that amount would go to Dr. Welch. For delivering that baby in the middle of the night, with almost a hundred miles of driving, he would have almost twenty dollars to spend. These mental gymnastics really woke him up.

He went into Dr. Welch's office after lunch the next day. He sat down, a man with a purpose, and declared, "Alex, we have a problem."

"We do?" the surprised Dr. Welch replied, showing a flicker of seldom seen emotion.

"Yes, we do. The new Burroughs machine has just uncovered it. I'm sure you have seen those printouts," he added.

"I thought they looked really good," Dr. Welch smiled. "Our incomes have risen dramatically. This new office is paying off, just as you predicted. I realize now I was wrong to fight you on that."

Malcolm remained calm as he continued, "I'm talking about the disparity of production. Yours is remarkably low."

"Harumph!" was his only response, but Alex was becoming noticeably uncomfortable.

"I know you have your way of doing things and I'm not critical of that, but the figures don't lie and we need to make some changes in our agreement. I propose we share the overhead on a percentage basis, not fifty-fifty. If I am bringing in 80% of the gross income…and I am, then I will pay 80% of the overhead, but we'll each take home our own money earned."

"Look here young man, I established this practice for many years before you came in," he responded with defensive anger, his heavily jowled face reddening rapidly.

"I realize that, Alex, but this is eleven years later. That is not a factor now. I did the math, and this year, so far, I am giving you $60,000 and it is only September. This has been going on for years and I didn't realize it. You have been treating Mayor Bixby and all of city hall for no charge as well as all your old, old friends like Buxton, who runs the service station. I charge everyone equally. I'm donating half of your largesse and you get all the credit. This is hurting my morale. I could ease off to your level of effort but I'm having too much fun. I'm just geared differently than you are."

Thinking to take a little of the sting out of his comments he added, "Sometimes I think you're smarter than I am in that regard."

"We're not changing anything." Dr. Welch was hurt and extremely agitated now.

"Just calm down Alex," Malcolm said carefully, "You need to think this over thoroughly and we'll talk again later."

Dr. Welch could not stop thinking it over. He was the established, senior partner. He would not be belittled by taking a lower salary. That upstart, McKenna, was more of a showman than he was a doctor. Who did he think he was? Just because he was good looking and attracted all those women…….Welch believed he was really the better doctor. Alex rationalized in every way possible before Dr. McKenna approached him a second time.

"Alex, we have a good thing going here. All we need to do is make some minor adjustments in the agreement. I've been thinking…and if you want us to have equal salaries that's fine. We can give the overage to a charity. I've been thinking about a foundation. The tax consequences are huge."

"Hold on……don't say another word. If you want to change our iron clad agreement, get a lawyer. I'm not discussing it further."

Malcolm was in total disbelief. How could anyone not see the problem? How could he be so set and stodgy?

"You're serious?"

"I am."

Malcolm stood up to leave. The room was rife with explosive animosity.

"I will get a lawyer and we will split this partnership."

Alex Welch had said aloud at that meeting what he had said silently from the very beginning.

"I don't need anyone. I'm the good guy here. Why do I let this neophyte run my office?"

Malcolm, the eternal optimist, was blinded by such thinking. He thought that down deep inside Dr. Welch was a good guy and he thought he was smart enough not to bite the hand that fed him.

He was wrong.

Chapter XIII

A Fight to the Finish

After that meeting, Malcolm knew he was in for a rough time. He was a realist when the chips were down. He plotted his strategy carefully. He read over their agreement and he saw immediately that all contingencies were covered for friendly separation like death, illness and the draft, but it was not spelled out who would get the office in a situation like this.

He naturally felt that it was his creation and his very survival depended on his ownership. He plotted a course to that end. He knew Dr. Welch's impulsive anger would be self-defeating. He would play the cat and mouse game. He would be the mouse and encourage Alex to be the cat. Alex was setting himself up for that game. He had rationalized himself into being the major player. Malcolm was well-suited to going back from the first time they met and sorting out Dr. Welch's weaknesses.

He would play the role of the naïve newcomer that Dr. Welch made him out to be. All the while he would work out a strategy to buy him out and own the office. He called his trusted high school friend, Bill Rose. Bill had gone into law while Malcolm pursued medicine. He had gone into practice with a major law firm in downtown Portland.

"Bill, I have a real battle on my hands. We're splitting the partnership and I'll need your help. I'm more than ready for the infighting if you make it legal."

"Sorry to hear that, Malcolm, what do you want me to do?"

"First I'll send you a copy of our agreement, which tells me the office is up for grabs. I want it. Tell me if I'm reading it right."

Four days later Alex was shocked to get a letter from Bill Rose stating that Dr. McKenna was quitting the partnership, but not the premises. He purposely did not make any claims as to building ownership. That letter set the stage for the two doctors to practice in the same office, beginning the next week.

Malcolm, who had always managed the office, had no trouble setting up his side of things but Alex was caught off guard. Reality set in immediately. He was the proverbial fish out of water. His problems would multiply during the nine months this situation was to endure. No one could foresee such a prolonged separation and Alex was at once taken aback by his plummeting income. He would really feel the hurt as time went on. The more he hurt the more angry he became and the frustration propelled him deeper into his well established rut. McKenna's flair and enthusiasm had, from the beginning, grated on Dr. Welch. Now he had the excuse to destroy him.

Dr. Welch's political connections would come into play. He spread the word to the state and county medical societies. He had always, as one might expect, followed their edicts. He easily fell in line because he lived the line. He was never comfortable away from the line. The line was magnetic for him. He was the exact opposite of Malcolm. The line is not between moral and immoral or right and wrong. The line is between innovative and status quo, between optimism and pessimism. Malcolm was 'straight arrow' to the core.

Dr. Welch carried his rumor crusade to all the city fathers to whom he had been giving free service. They were a tight knit group in this small town. The rumor mill sprang into action. Their purpose was to rid Stirling of this misfit. Malcolm had deeply offended one of their own. They were indignant and determined to see that he leave town. The very same people who had been telling Dr. Welch what a great doctor he had brought into town were now ready to tar and feather McKenna.

The wild tales about Malcolm's womanizing became more prevalent and specific. He suddenly was seen everywhere, drinking and living it up. He was planning a move to Hawaii, a better playground. He was moving to Hollywood and gambling in Las Vegas, the list of blatant debaucheries was endless. This wishful thinking would prove counter-productive to their cause. The Welch camp was lulled into a false sense of security.

Dr. McKenna visited Dr. Welch in his office in an attempt to counter this campaign of deceit.

"Alex, we are professionals and should be above all this trashy talk. I hope you will put a stop to it. These are your friends, so please take care of it."

Dr. Welch put forth his best smile and actually laughed out loud, something Malcolm had never seen before and stood up to signal the meeting had ended.

"So, McKenna, you're running scared."

Malcolm was dumbfounded. He couldn't imagine anyone being so blind to the reality of a situation. He stood close and looked squarely into Alex's cruel, accusing eyes. He looked into his very soul and he was sickened by what he saw there.

"I have only one thing to say to you and these will be my last words. I will never speak to you again………..I feel sorry for you."

He turned and left the room.

Malcolm worked harder than ever because the rumors brought more patients to his door. Most everyone wanted to get a glimpse of this superman. Even Malcolm, however, could not live up to what was being said about him. He worked and he planned.

He could have his pick of office personnel. His professionalism, work ethic and talent made them admire and respect him. He chose whom he wanted as his receptionist, nurses and bookkeeper. Dr. Welch would be well served in any event because Malcolm had hired all of them and they were good. The bookkeeper, Marielle, was especially talented. She was the front office manager. Her books were impeccable. She was honest to a fault. Her starched persona matched that of Dr. Welch. She carried a briefcase and she marched to her office daily, promptly at 8:00 a.m., like an automaton. The other girls respected, but hated her.

Because of her holier-than-thou airs, Malcolm did not choose Marielle. He knew she would be hard to replace but he wanted his girls to be happy. He was wise enough to know that contentment was key to efficiency. A happy group would want to keep up with the pace he set.

Shortly after the separation of the personnel was decided, Malcolm received a surprise visit to his office. Marielle seemed ill at ease sitting on the edge of her chair in front of his desk.

"Dr. McKenna, I was shocked when you didn't keep me. We have worked so well together. You must know how I respect you."

"Marielle, I fully understand where you are coming from. I respect you too. Your ability and performance are above reproach. You are a perfectionist, as a bookkeeper should be. I doubt that I can ever replace you…that's why I gave you to Dr. Welch, he will need you. You will call all the shots with him. You will replace me in that regard."

Marielle became even more uncomfortable. She fidgeted in her chair. She didn't know how to put into words what she had come to tell him.

"Dr. McKenna," she took a deep breath, "you must know that I love you. Oh, maybe you think it's all professionalism, but it's not……I love you as a man. You're the only man I've ever had such feelings for. You will have dedication, in every sense of the word, if you keep me," her eyes pleaded with him to change his mind.

Malcolm, who prided himself with understanding women, was taken by complete surprise. He saw it instantly now. Behind those horn-rimmed glasses and briefcase was a hot-blooded woman just waiting for the right moment to reveal herself. Now he was the uncomfortable one. What could he say? How could he say it and still be the kind-hearted person he was?

"Marielle…..you honor me. You………."

Marielle plunged right ahead, interrupting, "If you think that new nurse, Jill, is so desirable, just take another look at me….you'll find me more of a woman, in every way, than she could ever be."

Malcolm was shaken. He searched for words.

"Marielle, you have always amazed me, but this is beyond amazement. You, of all people, know that I don't really need anyone. You will be indispensable to Dr. Welch. I see a happy life ahead there for you. Keep him afloat so that I don't have to feel guilty. Will you do that for me?"

He stood up. They embraced. She knew he was right. Dr. Welch and her husband, they both needed her.

Malcolm, who had protected so many secrets, had one more to file away.

Chapter XIV

Jill Martin

Jill, the new nurse so hated by Marielle, had been interviewed by Dr. McKenna about a year before the split of the partnership. When he entered his office and saw her sitting there most of his questions were instantly answered without asking her a single thing.

He would hire her.

Trying hard not to find her flaws, he began, "Have you worked in a doctor's office?"

"No."

"Are you working now?"

"No."

"Have you worked in the last five years?"

"No."

"Why do you want to work now?"

"I'm getting a divorce."

He wanted to say 'you're hired.' Instinctively he knew this woman was as brilliant as she was beautiful.

At last he hit on the right question, even though it didn't apply to this job.

"Can you type?"

"Yes, 70 words a minute and I can take dictation in shorthand."

The interview was conducted during his lunch hour so he had time to find out what really made this captivating beauty tick. She was excused forty-five minutes later and told she would be contacted the following day.

Dr. Welch and Marielle had interviewed her earlier that morning but Malcolm did the hiring. Dr. Welch crossed paths with Dr. McKenna in his office that afternoon.

"What do you think of Jill Martin?"

"I don't know if she has a brain, but she sure as hell is good looking," Alex grinned.

"She does and a well-developed one at that. I'm going to hire her."

Malcolm was stunned to hear Alex say such a thing about a woman. He had never heard him make such a revealing comment regarding the opposite sex. It just wasn't Alex.

When Marielle was told of Malcolm's decision, her comment was brief.

"Look out…she's a black panther…."

Jill had lunch at her mother's house after the interview.

"Did you get the job?" her mother asked.

"I don't know yet. If it's up to the older doctor…maybe. If it's up to the bookkeeper…no. But if it's the younger doctor's call…yes, without a doubt."

It was his call.

She was in for many changes in her unhappy life.

* * *

You would notice Jill Martin in any setting. She was a statuesque brunette whose posture belied royalty. That façade could be a deterrent for the casual observer and her quick mind could be easily overlooked.

Malcolm saw it at the interview. He knew he could teach her everything an office nurse needed to know and do. He preferred inexperience over bad experience. Every procedure in medicine was sacred and he wanted it done his way. Detail was his forte, his stock in trade. Little things put together properly spelled diagnosis and from the nurses point of view…treatment.

Jill did not disappoint him. In a few weeks, she could draw blood, give injections and do lab work to his satisfaction. She quickly grew to have complete respect for this man. It would be safe to say she was in awe of him. To her, he was superhuman, untouchable. His close contact with her was controlled and professional and his knowledge and dexterity with medical procedures was flawless. With her it was always brains over brawn and this man was brilliant. She had also noticed that he was handsome. He had it all and she was not alone in her assessment, all of the girls in the office felt the same way about him.

Malcolm loved to help ladies in distress and he sensed that in her from the first day. He would talk to her in private about the divorce. He knew at once that she had married very young to a military uniform. He knew that two young children had prevented her from leaving an abusive relationship at an early date.

Jill was completely unaware that seemingly disconnected questions, on numerous brief encounters, were Dr. McKenna's prelude to a diagnosis. He was carefully assessing her plight and deciding how to help this "damsel in distress."

About four months into her tour of duty, she was leaning against the side counter of the front desk one morning, sharing some latest office tidbit with Wendy. Dr. McKenna walked up behind her and began talking to the receptionist too, about a new patient. His right hand rested on the counter top, holding a patient's chart, while out of view his left hand was making another statement to a startled Jill. He placed it firmly and openly against the middle of her lower back. Her muscles reflexively tightened. He felt her body, warm with the promise of things to come. She was taken completely by surprise as she read the statement correctly, "Jill, I want you and I always take what I want." She gripped the counter to absorb the unexpected implications of what had just occurred. As though nothing out of the ordinary had taken place, Malcolm walked away to see his next patient. The receptionist answered the phone unaware of the momentous event that had happened right before her unobservant eyes.

Jill's divorce troubles melted away as she went to bed that night with thoughts of Dr. McKenna foremost on her mind. She almost feared the power he could display with such nonchalance. Should she think of him as human now? She could hear her heart pounding at the very thought.

None of the girls had any inkling of what was on Malcolm's mind.

Jill knew…and that secret was almost more than she could bear.

She watched him continue seeing the patients day after day and began to feel she may have misinterpreted his gesture. Could it have been wishful thinking? The pattern of business as usual was broken the very next day when he asked her and two of the other nurses out to lunch. Jill was not as surprised as Molly and Meredith, who had worked there for years and had never seen this side of him before. He made it all seem businesslike when he questioned them about how to improve office procedure.

It was a fun lunch, however, and he showed his sense of humor when he read over the bill and asked in all seriousness, "Okay, which one of you ordered *spoo*?"

They all checked it out and concluded that it was a poorly written word for the *special*. Jill always remembered that lunch. She liked his fun side as well as his work ethic. She was finding many little things to like about him now that she had the freedom to engage in his flirtatious advances.

Dr. McKenna bought Beth a new Jaguar XKE for her birthday. It was delivered to the office to set the stage for a surprise appearance at the farm later that day. Jill and the office girls were in the parking lot looking it over when he walked out the door for lunch. He waited until everyone had returned to their posts and he grabbed Jill's arm as she started to go in.

"I want to give you a ride in this beautiful piece of machinery before its virginal smell dissipates."

She was impressed how he had sorted her out from the group so cleverly and easily.

"What a treat," she smiled as he opened the door for her.

They took a short drive on nearby winding roads and on their way back some unexpected words wrapped around her.

"I wish I could buy you one of these. You would look good in it. I really do admire you, you know. You're so comfortable to be with."

"You mean like an old shoe?" she teased.

"No, I mean more like a glass slipper. You could never be like an old shoe to me."

Those spontaneous, tender words would live in Jill's heart forever.

Beth and Malcolm were lying in bed one evening, in the quiet darkness. He was holding her hand to let the heat of her femininity course through his tired body.

"Beth, I need three or four wives," he said out of nowhere.

"I know," she answered.

"I'm serious. I have found number two."

"I'm serious too. I've always known that women are your weakness and your strength." She thought back five years when she had almost lost him to a Hollywood beauty. She was better prepared this time. "You should have all the wives you need as long as I am one of them. Tell me about this second wife," she added quietly.

He was totally unprepared for Beth's candor.

His silence prompted her to add, "Have you slept with her?"

"No, not yet."

Beth's answer, as usual, was a lingering kiss that ended the conversation and they went to sleep shortly thereafter.

Jill's second date with Malcolm took place about a week after their first group luncheon. He took her to a cozy spot much farther from the office.

There he questioned her at great length about her pending divorce. Her husband, Jake, had left the house at her insistence several weeks earlier but he had returned unexpectedly one night. He forced her to stand in front of him and strip. She really feared for her life after that episode in Texas when he put her in the car at gun point and marched her out on an isolated pier. She stood there for what seemed like hours, his finger on the trigger of the rifle that he held pointed in her direction. Now it was happening all over again. He taunted her, belittled her and called her vile names.

"You slut….You're giving it away…At least you should be paid for it. We could share all that money…."

Jill was crying as she confessed all these indignations.

Malcolm consoled her and promised an end to all this. He would put his lawyer on the case and they would get a restraining order.

"What kind of man could treat a woman like that? Well, that's easy," he answered himself, "the jealousy-ridden, hard-drinking, poor excuse for a man that she's divorcing."

She had been a virgin when they married. He was all she knew about men.

Jake was so self-conscious that he had never seen her nude until his recent unannounced visit. That fact explains how pathetic their life together really was. All their married years he had made love to her in the dark. She had so much to learn. Malcolm would cherish and protect her from this sordid past. She was motivated to experience his world that was so foreign to her.

Malcolm had detected the sadness in those beautiful eyes when they first met. He watched her now in amazement, this stately beauty rushing up and down the hall carrying such an unbelievable secret. She was magnificent. He needed her and she deserved the better life that he could give her.

Their third date, the magical one, would take place a few weeks later when he asked her to meet him after a medical meeting in Portland. The Chanticleer Restaurant was a perfect rendezvous. The basement lounge was candle-lit and far away from Stirling. Her face was even more hauntingly inviting in that dancing light. Glasses of Merlot teased their lips as they gazed into each other's eyes, unabashedly, for the first time. He wanted to taste that wine on her parted lips. He wanted to pour wine all over her and taste it.

He knew that he could not feel the way he did at this moment if she did not feel the same. What he didn't realize was that he had taken her, in his mind, as a second wife without her consent. She was having a hard time keeping up, so it was natural that she refused his invitation to a nearby motel.

"Do you always come on like gangbusters?"

He laughed out loud, "Only when I'm with you. This moment is sacred…….we shouldn't waste it."

"I'm sorry……I just can't do that," Jill looked away.

Alone in her bed that night she thought about Malcolm. She couldn't get him out of her head now. Was he too good to be true? If he wasn't, he had to be the smoothest operator she had ever come across. No, she thought, he was as sincere with her as he was with medicine. She had observed him day after day. He was real.

The fact that he was taken, haunted her. She knew she should back off. He was not available. He was not only married but married with five children. She didn't want to be involved with a married man. What had she gotten herself into? She drifted off to sleep, confused, but somehow happy about that rendezvous with Malcolm. His honest, straight forward approach was working its spell. His sincerity and persistence would overcome her innate fears about the unconventional world of this Saggitarian. He could carry her to the moon and points beyond.

Chapter XV

The Unfinished Business

Jill had worked at the clinic for almost three years when the partnership split happened. She and the other girls were not surprised. Dr. Welch always seemed like the person who got up on the wrong side of the bed. He was grumpy and sullen. His office door, located not far from their lunch room, was always closed. Every time they walked by, they thought of his personality…*closed* and *keep your distance*. Sometimes they wondered why he bothered with seeing patients or why patients bothered seeing him. The girls were unaware of all the *no charges* on the books that Dr. McKenna complained about during that fateful meeting.

The office was laid out beautifully, with the halls forming a large square around the central lab, x-ray and surgery. Each of the doctor's examination rooms branched off to the outside with opaque glass windows for good lighting. Dr. Welch was to the north and Dr. McKenna to the south. This separation and patient flow was ideal, especially now that the two were officially separated.

The girls often joked in private about the dark side and the bright side. Even though the work load was much heavier, they preferred to work with Dr. McKenna, who was always upbeat. His serious concentration inside the exam rooms never carried into the hall. They thoroughly enjoyed his jovial nature…the side he showed them.

The dark side became darker and the bright side even brighter. Lynne, who had been primarily Dr. Welch's nurse for years, was now in the enemy camp as far as McKenna's girls were concerned. All the office personnel were split into two groups now. This created a blanket of tension and incessant whispering was rampant.

One morning when Malcolm came into his office, about twenty

minutes before 8 a.m., he was met by a group of four of his girls. They stood, all in a row, with tears in their eyes. Wendy, the receptionist, was first to speak.

"We just can't stand to listen to all those lies that are being spread about you and in this very office, no less."

"Patients are so confused. Marielle leaves her back office and stands behind Wendy, harassing her, right out there where everybody can hear it. She's vicious," Brenda added with disgust.

The girls had never liked Marielle but now they literally hated her. Malcolm had foreseen problems with Marielle, that's why he did not include her on his list. He knew about the rumor war that Alex was perpetrating but he was a little surprised that the office was not off limits. He was both pleased and saddened that his girls were in front of him now. Pleased that they cared so much, but saddened by the scope of this outlandish crusade of lies. He chose his words carefully and with utmost sincerity.

"I know all about what is being said. I hate that it has come to this and I've tried, to no avail, to stop it at the source. I know who I am and you know who I am. That's all that matters. Rumors are like the leaves in fall, an attention getting brief entrance but they are predestined to rot on the ground. I appreciate your concerns, but don't feel sorry for us, feel sorry for them. They are the ones in trouble. By the way, don't any of you say one word, true or false, about Dr. Welch," he quickly added, "I'll fire anyone who does."

The girls left that meeting surprised, but reassured. They knew Dr. McKenna had his feet on the ground and would not be a pushover for anyone.

The office was the prize and he was preparing for that final meeting that would decide the issue. It had taken almost nine months. All the while he was healing the sick in a never ending stream. His girls were troopers and had their marching orders with that dramatic meeting. They worked harder and kept him so busy that he found it difficult at times to play "the mouse."

He did not lose sight of his game plan. He made trips to his bookkeeper's desk that was now shared with Marielle. He would whisper to his secretary and have her look up balances for him. He would look worried and leave. His acting perfectly portrayed a man with money problems. Marielle could be seen skittering down the hall to Dr. Welch's office, a short time later, carrying the secret.

His new bookkeeper, Faye, was a tough, bleached blonde perfectly selected to dish out as much brass as Marielle herself. Under these circumstances Malcolm knew that the small bookkeeper's office would be a powder keg. Faye more than held her own. She was a perfect plant. His strategy worked well and Dr. Welch licked his chops.

"I knew McKenna would fold without me. We'll have this office soon," he gloated to Marielle. "He's even afraid to be in the same room with me and the lawyers."

Because Malcolm lived up to his promise to never speak again to Alex, those meetings were short and productive. There was never any bickering.

Bill Rose would meet with Malcolm before each meeting and be instructed to come out with specific agreements. The first was Alex agreeing to allow Malcolm to have first pick on all the equipment and furnishings. Alex was to get equal value in the end. After all, the office was what he would fight for, not the contents. Malcolm would have to move out all that heavy stuff eventually.

The second meeting was all about accounting so it was easy for Malcolm to get what he wanted. He gave Bill Rose a written agreement to translate and formalize into legal terms. When such things as joint accounts, collection accounts and how to distribute patient records was presented, Dr. Welch *harrumphed* to cover his lack of knowledge and turned the whole thing over to his attorneys. Bill came away once again with Malcolm's wishes all bundled up legally.

It would be almost a month later when the granddaddy of all meetings took place. Who was to get the office? Malcolm had met with Bill several times to plot how to finesse that prize away from the cocksure Dr. Welch. The cat would now pounce and the mouse would be long gone. Malcolm explained to Bill how he was thought to be low on funds. He explained how that could work to their advantage in a put up or shut up cash deal. The partnership held two pieces of adjoining real estate. When the office lot was purchased by McKenna he had to buy three lots and houses and then trade for another lot to move one house onto. Then he traded that house for another lot near the office. Confusing, but necessary to show that the office carried with it some other commercially zoned real estate that Malcolm had plans for. It was natural, then, that he would tell Bill that the office included all that other property.

He wanted it to be a lump sum deal for two reasons. First, it made the buy-out figure much larger and secondly he had bigger plans for the future.

It was important to make the buy out figure a big number because he knew how afraid of borrowing Alex was. Malcolm knew that Alex would want to throw it all his way because Alex knew, or thought he knew, that McKenna was broke.

Alex may have had a plan to sell off parts and use his stand in with the city fathers to keep the office when McKenna couldn't comply with the put up or shut up approach. Bill played it to the hilt and seemed to shy away from the one stroke buy-out deal. Alex and his attorney pressured to lower the established buy-out figure, knowing Alex was the only one that could do it that way. McKenna would need some kind of a time payment deal for certain.

Finally, Alex, who was irritated by all this crazy talk, stood up and walked to the window. Malcolm had told Bill that he would do just that when he was worn down enough.

"Okay, it's settled then. McKenna will have to give me a cashier's check for $52,900 if he wants the office and it must close within the next five days." That figure was relatively large in those times, but it was well below the actual value of the property. Alex knew he could write such a check.

Bill looked ill at ease when he spoke, "That's a huge number, Dr. Welch. We'll write it up now and you sign it. I'll present it to Dr. McKenna tonight."

Bill's body language said that his client would be unable to perform.

After he left, Alex smiled and boasted, "We sure did outfox them this time, didn't we."

"I'm sure you'll get the office," agreed his lawyer.

Fearing a local bank mole, Malcolm had an account in Eugene where he had just sold some property. He had estimated the cost to be 30% higher. He smiled as he wrote the cashier's check. Now he owned the office.

* * *

The Dr. Welch crowd was stunned. They had only 90 days to move out with no place to move to. Dr. Welch was still trying to figure out what had happened. He never did.

Chapter XVI

Free to Fly with the Eagles

Malcolm was now cut loose from the grounding cables that a partnership entailed. He was his own boss at last. No one could use the gloom and doom argument every time he wanted the practice to grow and be more efficient. He was ecstatic. The reality of being all alone in such a large clinic was challenging, however. There would be no dark side in a few months, he would expand his efforts to fill the void.

Dr. Welch could never imagine such optimism. Through his eyes, McKenna was in for a fall. Somehow McKenna had won the first round but that would be his undoing. Dr. Welch thought he would return to the office before long. With that plan in place, he found a lot a few blocks away and set up his practice in two temporary mobile buildings. The move was costly and disorganized. That set-up was awkward and inefficient. The gross income dropped along with morale. Alex clung to the idea that a return to the established clinic would surely occur within six months or so. Marielle had free reign now and should have been very happy, but she was not pleased with the figures she had to work with. She longed for the old days and Dr. McKenna. She was a woman scorned so it was easy for her, after a while, to subdue those longings and replace them with Dr. Welch's hateful "destroy McKenna" plan.

Dr. Stacey was sought out by Dr. McKenna several months before the break up. The office had been built to accommodate a third doctor, explaining why Malcolm thought it would add to the efficiency of the clinic. The real reason he hired him, however, was to break up the two-man tie vote at management meetings. He was wrong, as it turned out, and much too late to be a factor in reducing the tension. Dr. Welch always attempted to control Malcolm with his wet blanket of pessimism.

When the split occurred, Malcolm did not ask Dr. Stacey to stay with him. He was not being magnanimous in this case, as he was with Marielle. Managing the office put Malcolm in a position to know the new doctor in a way completely unseen by Dr. Welch. It took only four months for Malcolm to know that as likable as John Stacey was, he was going to be a drag financially. His gross receipts were so low that time would not correct the fact that he would have to be supported. He was much more phlegmatic than Dr. Welch, who was not exactly overly ambitious.

Dr. Welch jumped at the chance to woo Dr. Stacey, knowing that to the outside it would look good for him to so isolate McKenna. Dr. Stacey would be a part of the so-called *Welch Crew*. Malcolm smiled inside knowing what an expensive partner he would be. Dr. Welch would be stuck with him because if he let him go, it would look bad. His "destroy McKenna" plan was already becoming very expensive. The cat had once again pounced to find the mouse long gone.

Playing the mouse game was almost too easy for Malcolm but he much preferred to enjoy his new found freedom and fly unfettered. First, he had long recognized a need at the MeRe Center. This center was a school for the mentally retarded run by the Episcopal Church. The mother of a long standing patient family was administrator there. He knew of their financial problems and his newly formed McKenna Foundation came to the rescue. His children had attended kindergarten there, the only private school in town. Another strong connection was Maria Sanchez, Father Bogarth's housekeeper and confidant, was also a long time patient. It will be important in events to follow, that you know of this strong connection to Father Bogarth.

The McKenna Foundation idea was born when he was talking to Dr. Welch and tried to solve their problems by suggesting that he would be open to the plan of equal take home salary. He had hoped that if both doctors were paid the same, in spite of their lopsided productivity, that Dr. Welch's ego problem would not interfere. Charitable donations could have been part of the imbalance. Of course, we know this did not solve Dr. Welch's indignities about the fact that he was the pioneer and the mainstay of their partnership.

This incident is important because it so typified Malcolm's kind and gentle nature. Almost everything reveals his lion heart but his hidden strong values were seldom so evident. On the time line, however, when he first found himself alone in that huge office building, his ideas about healing the sick expanded to fill the void. While the *Welch Crew* were treading water in their trailer encampment, salivating over his demise, he was dreaming of, and creating, a one-man medical clinic the likes of which had never been seen before or, I daresay, since.

The morale of his office crew was already very high because they had dodged the bullet of a disastrous move. Dr. McKenna's stature rose to new heights when they realized he had somehow pulled off a miracle. They would have been even more impressed had they known the details and the odds. They didn't. He didn't want them to ever know that he had portrayed himself as a mouse. Malcolm capitalized on his elite staff, so inspired by recent events.

"From this day forward no patient will be turned away by rescheduling. If they feel they need to be seen that day, we will work them in. I will always be here at 8:00 a.m. and I will stay through the noon hour if need be, but we will always leave as close to 5:00 p.m. as possible. You get them into a room, and we do have plenty of those now, and I will see them. I want the time they arrive up in the right hand corner of each work sheet that is attached to the chart. No one should wait longer than thirty minutes. Our goal will be fifteen minutes."

His receptionist, Wendy, commented as he paused for a breath. "Doctor, that's a very tall order, what if……."

Dr. McKenna interrupted, "There will be rare exceptions to any rule, but we'll discuss those over weekly meetings in the lunch room. I plan to bring my lunch and eat there from now on. I hope you won't mind?"

"I have an idea," Lucy, the quiet little front office worker spoke up, wanting to help out. "We could take turns fixing lunches if the doctor doesn't mind footing the bill, that way many of us will be available for emergencies."

"You girls talk that one over. If you decide to act on Lucy's suggestion, I certainly will pay for the food."

He instructed Faye, his new bookkeeper, to set up an account that would pay for grocery receipts brought to her.

As it turned out, those lunches were a big success. The girls socialized more and brought up office procedural problems. They began bringing casserole dishes from home and enjoyed the positive feedback. Malcolm was too busy to partake most of the time but he did make it a point to have a short weekly meeting at least. The girls felt even closer to him when he heard their suggestions.

The momentum shifted more and more to high morale and efficiency. It became a game with them to see if they could keep him so busy that at some point he would have to cry "uncle." An unusual and funny incident that occurred a few years later would illustrate this point.

It was 5:15 p.m., on a Friday, after a very busy day and week. The girls decided to make Dr. McKenna aware of how exhausted they were and he should be. The last patient had left the building and he was walking down the hall, chart in hand, toward his office, where a huge pile of charts was waiting on his desk. He always wrote on them in his office when a convenient break occurred because he wanted to look the patient in the eye when he talked to them. He did not want that relationship disturbed by writing. He wrote all of his notes long hand to personalize them and make them more accurate. No dictation here, except for letters to doctors and lawyers.

He had a photographic memory that allowed him to make the notes hours after the events. In his mind he would recreate the scene, including what was said and what the examination showed. He always put down a working diagnosis and treatment. He would even write notes to himself in the left margin to include personal things like, "They just got a new black lab puppy named Bart" or "Grandma Effie from West Virginia is coming to live with them."

Patients were usually astounded when he walked in the room for an office visit a year later and casually asked about Bart or Grandma Effie. He then had the patient instantly in a proper mood to talk (and quickly reveal their diagnosis). Malcolm's ability to read extra verbal and verbal communications was a science and an art. He was focused at all times but appeared to be so friendly and relaxed. He would always sit down when he talked to his patient. The patient always left the office properly treated after a five minute visit that seemed to them an hour. If a problem was very complex, he scheduled them for a complete physical later when more time was available. He seemed to be blessed with a sixth sense.

The girls had planned their stunt so carefully that they knew he would be impressed and have to acknowledge their flawless work ethic. When he approached his office, ten girls were propped up against the walls and sprawled over his carpeted office floor. They were *exhaustion* spelled out plainly and in no uncertain terms.

He pondered the chart in his hands as he stepped around and over them, one by one. He seated himself at his desk and proceeded with his writing. He appeared to have seen nothing. Finally, they all jumped up and laughed out loud. He laughed with them. He so admired their esprit de corps, but thought, rightly so, that he honored them more when their joke became his joke.

The girls envied Dr. McKenna's boundless energy. He was always up and never missed a day due to illness. Stimulants were certainly not the answer. He treated his body with utmost respect and never drank or smoked. His weight remained constant even though he loved to eat. He always had a garden and raised all of his own meat on his farm.

The office continued to evolve as he hired more help to keep up with the growing patient load. It ended up that he employed two receptionists, four front office girls including the head bookkeeper, and four nurses in the back, one of whom was Jill Martin.

These nurses were multi-talented. They took x-rays and did lab work, including EKGs. All had been trained by Dr. McKenna to do things his way. He wanted perfection and that's what he got. All new hires were on a conditional three-month basis.

If he had to let them go he would say, "I'm sure you'll do fine in most any other office, but you are aware now of what a pressure cooker this is."

The receptionist's job was one of the most difficult to fill. The nurses loved their jobs and their doctor so much, they seldom left.

The receptionist had to be Miss Congeniality. She was expected to put a happy, caring face on the office. The telephone and charts were her constant distraction. McKenna's hand was felt in every faction of his operation.

"There's good stress and bad stress but all we have here is good stress," he would say, "Patient's who are ill always come in grouchy but must leave in good spirits. That's our job and our reward."

His attitude was contagious and the office reeked of it. Patients noticed.

This office metamorphosis would have been remarkable under normal circumstances but the venom spread by Dr. Welch did not let up. In fact, the more Dr. McKenna accomplished, the more his enemies plotted to destroy him. Dr. Welch finally, after about two years, decided he was not going to be able to return to the clinic building. He had to start construction on his own office. This added even more fuel to the fire that burned inside him. Financial stress was taking its toll all the while. He plotted with his county medical society cronies and they were quick to agree that Dr. McKenna's methods must be suspect. He did not fit any mold they knew; he had to be controlled at all costs. Envy continued to fuel the fire. A witch hunt was born.

Chapter XVII

A Balancing Act

In Malcolm's mind he already had a second wife….Jill. Beth, wife number one, knew about it long before Jill was convinced. This situation created some interesting interludes.

"I got a call from someone today about you," Beth smiled.

"What are you talking about?" He wondered what was going on now.

"The caller said you were having an affair with Jill Martin."

"And what did you say?"

"I said thank you for telling me but it is not really an affair."

"That must have confused the caller. Who was it, by the way?"

"I don't know who it was, but he did seem a little disappointed when he hung up. I do think he had hoped to make trouble for you."

"I'm not at all surprised. It doesn't really matter who it was but I appreciate your response. I'm sure it deflated his balloon." He smiled at Beth, "By the way, what's for dinner"

"Your favorite, macaroni and cheese," she said sweetly. "And if you don't mind my asking, how are you and Jill getting along these days?"

"She's having a hard time adjusting but it will work out given a little time," he said confidently.

He let that settle for a moment before adding, "And, by the way, in case you're wondering, I haven't committed adultery as your mystery caller implied. We need to have a discussion about that some time when food is not getting cold."

They kissed and she served him his late supper. On his way to the office early the next day, he pondered the full meaning of that call to Beth. He knew all about the forces being brought to bear against him by Dr. Welch but he seldom gave it all that much thought. He was too busy creating a positive protective universe in the center of which he was untouchable by such malcontents as that caller. Beth had unknowingly thrown cold water on some well thought out skullduggery.

"Curses, foiled again." In his mind he named the caller Simon Legree.

With his help Jill had rid herself of that awful, oppressive marriage. She was more beautiful than ever, a joy to behold. He was with her in those halls at the office every day. So close and yet so untouchable, their attraction to each other fomented. Work was the damper that made it bearable. To the other girls and the patients those magnetic forces between them went unnoticed. This was professionalism of the highest order. Together they went about the business of caring for the ill.

Beth was the beneficiary of such frustration. Malcolm felt a warm release in her arms and her kisses. They had grown apart in so many ways. He felt like he had six children to come home to and not five. She was in no way lacking in the IQ department, but she just somehow could not connect with his dreams and aspirations. She loved her home life, she loved her children and her mind stayed in that world. Her basic desires carried over into the bedroom.

Jill had met the Malcolm that Beth never knew. She fell in love with the dreamer, the man with full fledged wings. Beth had known and married the little boy, Malcolm, whose wings were forming inside and waiting to sprout. Jill was an artistic, right-brained dreamer herself. She could better understand the practical left-brained Malcolm. He was complex, but so was she. Together they possessed a matched set of right and left brains. Together they would be awesome.

Malcolm pondered this conundrum of two women equaling one wife. The law was blind to such a possibility he concluded. What to do? He knew that honesty always was the best policy to prevent tangled webs. It all jelled in his mind and he spoke to Beth in bed early one morning.

"The way it turns out, I cannot legally have two wives but deep down I knew that all along. However, if I'm not married I can legally have two mistresses."

"Are you still fretting this thing? I told you several weeks ago that you can have four wives as long as I'm one of them."

"You don't understand Beth, the law and marriage can make me an adulterer. If I'm single, the law does not apply, right?"

"You've lost me on that one. What more can I do than share you with another woman?"

"You can divorce me," he said in all seriousness.

"What?" Beth was stunned by this turn of events.

"I said we can get a divorce that no one will know about. Just you and I will know and I can have the two of you legally."

At first Beth thought he was joking but now she knew he was deadly serious with this proposition.

"I don't know….this sounds too strange to me."

Malcolm continued, "There is another benefit to divorce."

Trying to sell this new idea he said, "The practical side comes into play here. Our income taxes will go down considerably. There's a thing called the marriage penalty. I didn't know it existed but it does. Crazy, huh?"

"It sounds as though this is not just a passing thought. You're really serious, aren't you?"

"Absolutely. I plan to get Bill Rose on it right away. Okay?" Malcolm couldn't hide the excitement in his voice.

"It doesn't sound like I have any choice and I'll do whatever you want anyway, you know that, but at least let me think this over for a while."

A few weeks of talks finally convinced Beth and she reluctantly agreed to his proposal.

Bill Rose worked his magic and a few months later that certificate of marriage, long ago lost in some drawer, no longer existed. No one knew where it was when it was valid and no one knew it had been invalidated.

Finally Malcolm felt free to fulfill his dream of having two wives. A double life, with all the intrigue it would entail, appealed to him. He told Jill that he was no longer married. She was dumbfounded. She had no idea what he had been up to but this news delighted and excited her. He told her that it was a secret not to be revealed. He also told her that he would never, under any circumstances, marry again. Jill had to think this turn of events over very carefully. The next day she spoke her mind.

"Malcolm, I haven't made any secret about how much you mean to me and although this is not the ideal arrangement, I can't imagine my life without you in it. That said, I will accept you on your terms and I will love you completely and unreservedly from this day forward."

"Jill, I'm so in love with you, how could I not be?"

They embraced and sealed the bargain with a lingering kiss.

Almost a week later, on a Saturday afternoon, they consummated their love in a rustic little cabin in the foothills of Mt. Hood. What had been so anticipated was such a powerful release of pent up desire that they slept peacefully in each other's arms until after midnight.

His double life had begun.

Jill had more of his time than Beth, but not as a husband. Hers was the professional relationship. She enjoyed this untouchable side of him but their intimate time was clandestine and awkward.

No one, including her two children, would know their secret. He could not see her in her home or in the close environment of Stirling. She awkwardly slid down to the floorboard, with her long legs cramped beneath her, to be out of sight if they traveled through areas where they might be recognized. Usually they met in the big city where they could get lost together.

The movie classic, Dr. Zhivago, premiered at the Paramount Theatre in Portland at this time. They were looking for excuses to get lost and this movie sounded ideal. It was a tragic love story between Zhivago, played by Omar Shariff, and Julie Christie, who portrayed Lara, the nurse. Their love was thwarted throughout the movie by the 1917 Russian Revolution. It ended when he finally returned, gray-haired and physically weakened by his forced war service. He discovered she had moved from the upstairs hide away apartment where they had always met.

The passing years added to his frailty and he looked tired as he stared from the window of the city bus on that fateful day. He was suddenly startled to consciousness when he spotted Lara, walking alone across the street. He jumped to his feet, his heart pounding, as he hurried to the front of the bus where he implored the driver to stop. He ran to find his long lost love. Suddenly he was stopped in mid-stride by a jolt of excruciating pain and clutching his chest, he fell lifeless to the ground. *Lara's Theme* was the haunting song that played throughout this emotionally charged movie. Dr. McKenna and Jill identified so completely with what they were watching that they left their bodies sitting in the darkness, holding hands, with tears flowing profusely. They were Julie Christie and Omar Shariff.

Arm in arm they supported each other as they walked from the theatre in a blissful state of exhaustion. *Lara's Theme* became their song. It would always transport them back to that time when their love was so inspired.

* * *

As the years went by, Jill longed for an open relationship but she never voiced her feelings to him. She was incredibly patient and stoic.

Beth obviously was wrought with mental anguish from time to time, knowing he was with the other woman. He was home most evenings and therefore all family events and holidays. He had always been away so much on hospital and house calls, as well as medical meetings, that even his children were not suspicious. Beth kept the secret to herself. In this regard, both Jill and Beth deserved medals. He was fully aware of their sacrifices and was touched by such loyalty.

The strong point of this triangle was that it required an undercurrent of competition between the two women. They both wanted to please him. His rewards were numerous but he paid a heavy price, being in two separate worlds all the time required superhuman effort.

Here it should be repeated that medicine is a jealous mistress. In reality, he was torn in three, not two, directions. Medicine always came first, both Beth and Jill were at peace with that.

Jill, who participated directly in that part of Malcolm's life, had some advantage. The strong family ties favored Beth. The reality of it was that he had created more "good stress," as he liked to think of it, than even he could handle easily.

On occasion he had to eat two Thanksgiving dinners. He, at times, would be thinking about a problem in one of his worlds, while living in the other. Neither Jill nor Beth ever knew of these distractions, however. Most of his problems were with medicine, and practicing in the hostile environment still alive and well under the direction of his old partner, the bitter, vengeful Dr. Welch. The local city fathers and the state and county medical societies were relentless.

The local group was annoying, but not lethal. They pecked away with rumors, first in the community college, where Malcolm was on the board and had become chairman of the medical department. He created and guided the classes for training office personnel. A summit meeting with Sue Bronson, a nurse who headed that department, and all the local office managers was held one Thursday afternoon in the fall of 1972.

Marielle, Dr. Welch's representative, was in attendance. The matter under discussion involved payment to office interns.

"Internships learning curve is indirectly proportionate to payment received…the lower the pay, the higher the learning benefits. It costs doctors to participate in this program and we should not expect them to pay for the inconvenience," Dr. McKenna proclaimed from the head of the table in answer to Sue Bronson's pitch for payment. She was carrying a liberal banner to protect her trainees.

The wisdom of his statement slowly sank in and a vote in agreement carried the day. Marielle sought out Dr. McKenna after the meeting.

"Now I know what makes you so invincible," she said acknowledging his victory over the battle for the office and his subsequent survival in spite of her camp's vendetta.

"Thanks for the compliment, Marielle, coming from you that means a lot to me," he replied, fully appreciating all the undercurrents.

* * *

A good example of how trite and desperate Dr. Welch's town spies were, is the barber shop incident. Malcolm was getting his hair cut in the local shop late one Friday afternoon. By chance, a reporter for the local weekly paper was in line. He asked permission to take a photo of the lady barber and her client for an article he was writing in his *Man About Town* column. Everyone involved was cordial and it all seemed innocent enough at the time. That photo, along with another of Dr. McKenna giving a talk about medical hypnosis at the local Kiwanis Club luncheon, somehow found their way into the county medical society. Due to a picture of Dr. McKenna in the barber's chair and that photo from the Kiwanis lecture, the medial society accused him of *advertising*...an ethics violation.

The witch hunt continued.

Chapter XVIII

Medical Hypnosis, a New Dimension

Dr. McKenna had always been frustrated by the fact that many illnesses he had to deal with had no specific treatment. Stress related problems such as headache and irritable bowel syndrome were prevalent. He knew that writing prescriptions for tranquilizers was easy but unsatisfactory in the long run. He, in no way, wanted to contribute to a doctor induced drug culture. He used reassurance whenever he could. Even though he was close to his patients, telling someone, "it's all in your head," is difficult.

When a brochure about medical hypnosis crossed his desk, shortly after the partnership split, he threw it in the waste basket along with all his other junk mail. He laughed at the absurdity of such an idea. He awoke the following morning trying to corral a thought rattling around in his head.

"I wonder if hypnosis really is a way to dial into the mind quickly and thereby better communicate?" That thought haunted him. A few weeks later brought another brochure advertising a meeting on medical hypnosis in Las Vegas.

"I need a break and Vegas sounds really good about now. What do I have to lose? I know I can spot the quackery in all this and then I'll be able to put it out of my mind and forget about it once and for all," he thought to himself. He signed up for the seminar. It would help satisfy his need for post graduate hours to accommodate his American Family Practice Academy membership, if nothing else.

At first glance, the main speaker, William Bryant, M.D., who practiced in Los Angeles, and was president of the American Hypnosis Society, had all the trappings of a charlatan.

"Part of that Hollywood crowd.......what have I gotten myself into here?" Malcolm smiled to himself. "This will be ridiculous, but entertaining, perhaps."

When Dr. Bryant spoke, first listing the conditions he had treated successfully, Dr. McKenna sat upright and listened intently. Dr. Bryant defined hypnosis as a method whereby one could hone in to the subconscious mind.

"It is a state of extreme concentration on the subject; a normal state that one passes through quickly going to sleep and awakening. We can hold that area of thought much as you can hold one frame in a motion picture. We can then talk to it and implant messages there. These will not be forgotten as they would be with the conscious mind."

Dr. McKenna maintained a healthy skepticism but he knew if this was genuine, it could revolutionize his practice. He could treat all those people who were falling through the cracks. He left Las Vegas excited to learn more.

He didn't have long to wait because soon a weekend workshop was held in Portland, sponsored by the Oregon Hypnosis Society, a fledgling group with no M.D. members at that time. Dennis Erickson, M.D., who was, interestingly enough, wheelchair bound was the main speaker. A practicing psychiatrist from Denver, Colorado, his credentials were impeccable. Dr. McKenna latched on to his fascinating mind and implanted it into his own. He came away, not only a believer, but a born again, card-carrying hypnotist. He was one of the first medical doctors to join the local and national societies to stay on the learning curve. He did not advertise his new skills other than to add the framed certificate of society membership to the wall in his office.

He now had a new leaf in his prescription pad; four weekly 1 hour sessions, on the new comfortable recliner in the corner of his private office filling another void in his treatment protocol. He usually had to have these sessions scheduled during the noon hour so that his regular schedule could accommodate them. This became a small, but indispensable part of his busy practice. It did, ironically, save him time when he became proficient in hypno-anesthesia.

He was called to the hospital one morning to treat a shoulder dislocation. When he walked into the x-ray room, the young basketball player was still on the table. The x-ray tech wanted to be sure his films were satisfactory before the patient was moved. Dr. McKenna went into the viewing room next door and studied them.

"Good pictures. I'll go and examine the patient then we'll see what needs to be done," he said aloud.

The tech was busy sorting films and did not follow him or he would have been truly amazed to see the five-minute shoulder reduction done under hypnosis. Usually, these cases were taken to surgery and reduced under the relaxation of general anesthesia.

Dr. McKenna suggested to the patient that the shoulder was packed in ice. Under hypnosis, the boy saw that happen. His shoulder became immediately cold to the touch and the dislocation was reduced instantly and painlessly. The doctor then poked his head in the viewer room door.

"Okay, Pete, you can take another film now."

"I thought you said the films were good."

"I did, but I want post-reduction films now," Dr. McKenna replied, to clear up his confusion.

Pete was perplexed and thought he somehow had misunderstood the order but he followed it anyway. He looked over Dr. McKenna's shoulder as he compared the films.

"There, looks good, doesn't it?"

"It sure does Doc, but how did you do that? His left shoulder was as cold as ice when I lifted him to place the cassette."

"It's called hypno-anesthesia. I've been using it lately to save time and expense to the patient."

After Dr. McKenna left for his office, Pete pondered the event he had witnessed. "I'll be damned…hypno-anesthesia. I've seen everything now. Dr. McKenna has always been a practical guy. He is amazingly practical."

Dr. McKenna reduced fractures and dislocations on his own x-ray table saving time and money for hospital admissions. He also used this method for hospital deliveries and because of it the infants were alert and pink; no more Apgar-9 blue babies.

* * *

Hillary Smith brought Brian, her four year old, in for a lingering cold.

"I find nothing to worry about, Hillary, Brian's chest is clear as is his nose and throat. It's viral. We'll watch him. Let me know if he's not well in a week."

"Doctor, I have a question about me. My husband is all upset because Brian is an only child. He wants me to have another baby."

"That's understandable, what do you want?"

"I would like another child too, but I'm so afraid of childbirth. My first delivery was in Spokane and it was a disaster."

"A disaster? Tell me what that means, Hillary."

Hillary began, "My regular doctor was unavailable when I went into labor. I was scared to death. The stand-in doctor tried to help, but everything that could go wrong, did. I had to get a transfusion of two pints of blood. All in all, I just can't do that again." She hesitated for a moment, then continued carefully, "I understand you do deliveries with hypnosis, do you think that would help me face this dilemma?"

"I sure do, Hillary, I'd be willing to give it a try if you will."

Hillary had always had a great respect for Dr. McKenna. She thought nothing was beyond his ability; she trusted him implicitly. About three months later, she came in pregnant.

"I'm really pleased you are going to have another baby, Hillary. I think it will solve a lot of your marital problems. After we schedule you for your O.B. physical we'll set up the hypnosis sessions. You know, the more intelligent the person, the better the subject, and you are certainly that. I'll teach you how to relax like you never have before."

True to his prediction, Hillary was so motivated to succeed, that she was very soon able to go into stage IV trance states, perfect for deep hypno-anesthesia. About six months into her pregnancy, she had to go to her dentist and was always full of fear there too. Dr. McKenna put her under and gave specific suggestions as to how she would completely relax, instantly, in the dental chair and how her face and jaw would be totally numb. A couple of weeks later he ran into her dentist on the street.

"What did you do to Hillary? I used to hate to see her come in, she was always so full of fear. This time, she literally collapsed in the chair. It frightened me for a few minutes, I had to check her pulse and blood pressure, but it was fine. Whatever you did, McKenna, I'm impressed."

"Hypno-anesthesia, Charles, it's a good short cut….if those non-believers only knew."

Hillary delivered a little girl a few months later. It was a breeze. Another drugless happy event. To make a point, Dr. McKenna told the nurse to get Hillary up off the table and give her the baby to carry out to show her worried husband. The nurse was certain the patient would collapse, and hesitated.

"I'll take all the responsibility, Fran, get her up," he ordered.

Hillary was all smiles and confident as she presented their beautiful new daughter to her husband. The nurses were amazed and impressed.

"What a change from last time. Doc, I owe you more than this cigar," her grateful husband said, barely able to control the emotion in his voice.

"I'm glad you got your girl, Frank. The pleasure was all mine. Congratulations."

Hillary was such an attractive and successful model for hypno-anesthesia, Dr. McKenna frequently asked her to come along for his talks about the misunderstood science of hypnosis.

It was at one such meeting that a picture was taken for the newspaper. It ended up in his medical society file, along with the fateful haircut clipping. Toeing the line did not include hypnosis. That was quackery. They knew of no other doctor using such an unproven method.

But, use it he did. Day after day. It saved him time and allowed him to write fewer prescriptions, always his goal. He was suspect of all new untried drugs and waited for them to be proven to his satisfaction, before using them. Many were pulled off the market in due time giving credence to his careful actions. He lived by the words of one of his pharmacology professors spoken so many years ago. *First of all, do no harm.* Iatrogenic deaths were never attributed to Malcolm because of the quote. Side effects always weighed heavy on that scale.

Patients began showing up from all over the state and a few from other states because of his success with hypno-therapy. He treated fears, phobias and bad habits, like smoking. He was honored to become the chairman for the American Cancer Quit Clinic for the county because of his successful ablation of cigarette smoking. He had always hated what smoking did to people, including his own father, who started the habit at age eleven.

It was a sunny afternoon and a perfect day for the football game between U of O, his alma mater, and Air Force, in Multnomah Stadium in Portland. He sat to the right of his father in the bleacher seats on the east side of the field. The players were running back into their locker rooms after their warm-up, when his father spoke, "Malcolm, you're no damned good when you get old."

A few seconds later he fell dead of a massive heart attack. Malcolm caught him, protecting the fan seated below. He had to drive home alone and tell his mother. That was very traumatic but he was always glad that he had been the witness rather than his mother. He knew what a blessing such an unexpected sudden death could be, he had seen so many prolonged illnesses involving pain.

He knew his father was programmed to live to be 90, but cigarettes shortened that by at least ten years, statistically speaking. He would continue to attack the cigarette menace with renewed purpose. Every patient he treated was diplomatically lectured if they were a smoker. Hypnosis was a reliable back up in this regard.

On one occasion, the steady flow of aches, pains and fevers, was happily interrupted by an out of state, attractive young lady complaining of stage fright and a mental block to mastering the German language.

"Doctor, I've heard about your skills with hypnosis and I wonder if you could help me?"

"I have never attempted to treat an opera singer with such problems, I must confess. Yours is definitely a problem of concentration. I would be surprised if hypnosis would not be the answer. We can certainly give it a try."

At the beginning of her third session, the patient offered some feedback as to her progress. "My voice instructor, in Seattle, said that my voice has improved more in the last week than at any time in the last year. He was unaware of my visits with you."

"Vocal cords respond to relaxation just like every other function of the human body. I'm happy to hear you are doing so well," he said encouragingly, "Now let's see what we can do about your upcoming audition in New York."

Malcolm's appreciation of the dramatic helped him with this case when he arranged for her to contact him by telephone, from her hotel room, just before the audition for the Metropolitan Opera in New York. They were duly impressed with her talent and she was hired on the spot. No one, except she and her doctor, knew that she was hypnotized for the event. Auditions were her nemesis, once past that point, her nervousness disappeared completely.

Hypnosis, Malcolm had found, was the key to unlocking the mind's control over illness. He used it judiciously and carefully. When would the medical world be ready to accept his realistic dreams?

Chapter XIX

A Lonely Road

Contrary to Medical Society thinking, he knew that medicine was not an exact science. The rank and file could be unchallenged and comfortable by adhering to the thought that treatment of disease was a kind of democracy. What was, in a sense, a majority rule consensus, was acceptable and anything else was suspect. The problem with that approach was that it was too slow to react to change or discovery. Malcolm, himself, saw the wisdom in going slow with new drugs but he parted company when new methods were not properly evaluated. He knew it was a fine line, indeed, that separated quackery from the cutting edge. He never crossed that line, but the casual observer would misunderstand him.

He stood alone in many of his treatments. Hypnosis is just one example. There were many, including Dr. Welch and the Medical Society, who wanted him to fail. The reason he survived is that his results were so amazing. Most consultants respected him and placed him in the "one of a kind" column. Some, who did not know him well, almost feared his blatant honesty and his "she bear" protection of his patients.

The surgical consult, Dr. Carter, who had operated on the four month old Holmes baby, and spoke so highly of McKenna, was a long time advocate of his. The same could be said of his associate, Dr. Halvorson.

Ned O'Brien, an 82-year-old, long time patient, was admitted to Stirling General by Dr. McKenna, with a working diagnosis of diverticulitis. Knowing that a ruptured diverticulum can be as fatal as an appendix, he called in the surgical consult, Dr. Halvorson.

"It will be later, after office hours, before I can see him, Malcolm. Is that okay?"

"Fine with me. I just don't want to overlook a rupture. Hard to tell in this old man, as you know. His white count is normal."

In this small hospital it was necessary to give a one hour lead time for non-emergency surgery after hours. Anesthesia and surgical nurses had to be called in. Dr. Halvorson followed this procedure and scheduled surgery before he called Dr. McKenna. It was about 7:30 p.m. when he reached him at home.

"Malcolm, I've scheduled surgery for 8:30 tonight on Mr. O'Brien. I expect you to scrub in as my assistant, okay?"

"I have one question, George. Why are we operating?"

After a long, awkward silence, Dr. Halvorson replied. "I………well……….he…Damn it, Malcolm, why did you ask that question? But I see your point. Let's watch him and get another count in the morning."

A big time consultant, from Portland, had put himself in a spot when he had to send the surgical crew home and cancel. He did just that, and his humility was not lost on Dr. McKenna. He admired him anew and that feeling was mutual.

The decision not to operate proved fortunate when Mr. O'Brien suffered a heart attack about 4 a.m. His diverticulitis and coronary occlusion responded to conservative therapy and he was discharged ten days later.

Another prime example of Dr. McKenna protecting his patient, took place a few months later at Providence Hospital in Portland. John Edwards was referred to an orthopedist for spinal surgery. Dr. McKenna did not usually assist on such cases in a Portland hospital. Mr. Edwards, one of Dr. McKenna's first patients in the fifties, had so much faith in his doctor, that he spoke up and surprised Dr. McKenna.

"Doc, I just don't feel like going under without you there. Would you?"

Dr. McKenna was flattered but knew it was not prudent, time-wise, to accommodate John Edwards.

"If you feel that strongly about this, I'll be there, John."

He was there, an hour before surgery, doing a pre-op appraisal of the patient. What he discovered astounded him. The anesthesiologist was prepared to give him a spinal block with the very drug that had almost killed John on a previous admission. Dr. McKenna consulted with the anesthesia department on the QT. He took it in stride that he had averted a catastrophe.

"Somebody has to keep track of the little things," he often reminded himself and his office help. He insisted that all drug allergies be written in red on the outside cover of each patient's chart. He also instructed his nurses that before any injection was administered, she should ask the patient about allergy to whatever drug was in the syringe. He kept careful track of the big picture while reveling in minutia. That undoubtedly accounted for the fact that he never had to defend himself in a lawsuit. This very same fact perplexed the Medical Society, whose in line M.D.s had all those problems. There was one, in their own highest echelon, who had three suits pending at one time. "Could it be that politicians have less time to devote to those 'little things'?" McKenna muttered under his breath. He had no time for politics.

Malcolm read the events unfolding around him like proverbial tea leaves. He had the kind of memory that put things on the back burner, to be brought forward at a later date, when appropriate, creating many "Eureka" moments. These definitely affected how he practiced medicine and perplexed the onlooker.

He gave a great many injectable medicines, not to make money, which he certainly didn't need, but to effect cures. To wit, Penicillin. He never forgot that case of pneumococcic meningitis from internship. You may recall how a chief resident berated him over that case. The resident had totally under rated Malcolm's prowess in diagnosis and treatment even then, when he was just a lowly intern. That resident had paid a heavy price for underestimating this fledgling M.D. It is ironic, that through the ensuing years, so many more would make the same mistake.

A point about Penicillin must be made here because it demonstrates so clearly how his mind catalogued and retrieved the past. The derelict alcoholic, found comatose in his apartment after five days, should not have survived. The interns in emergency, who sent him up to the contagious disease ward, had written a note defining his condition as moribund. He was given then unheard of doses of Penicillin, intravenously. He survived. Why? Because, not only was the meningitis correctly diagnosed, but the bug causing it was pinpointed promptly. This fact was the key to flooding the patient's blood stream with the exact antidote, so to speak. Penicillin. This was not a miracle but pure science, meticulously applied.

In light of this history, Dr. McKenna gave Penicillin by injection only. He knew that Penicillin was bacteriocidal, meaning that it directly killed bacteria. He wanted to be sure that the blood stream had high enough levels to sterilize it. That fact would not allow any bacteria time to develop resistance to the drug. When oral Penicillin is used a slower and incomplete action is the outcome.

Another problem with the oral route is that the stomach and intestines destroy most of the dosage. It never reaches the blood stream at all. Babies usually fight the spooned drug that has to be given at four hour intervals. A great deal of it is spit out and wasted, not to mention the night time interruption. One injection can last seven to ten days and give a constant high blood level.

Dr. McKenna so religiously followed his protocol that he, on occasion, turned away over protective mothers who refused to have their babies injected. It was literally impossible to educate a hysterical mother about these facts. When they insisted on drops, he simply said, "I will not be responsible for inadequate treatment that can have far reaching consequences. If you don't trust my judgment in this, please find a doctor who will compromise for you."

Most were shocked into listening, but a few did find a doctor who would cater to them. Those were politically correct practitioners who thought that shots were time consuming and painful. They rationalized that injections were only used by fringe M.D.s, out to make more money. Their own admission about time and effort involved nullified that assumption.

Dr. McKenna has been proven to be ahead of his time in the use of antibiotics. Thirty years later, resistant organisms present a huge problem. Many deaths are attributed to those "smart bugs". We have only seen the tip of that iceberg. Such deaths will reach pandemic proportions. Short sightedness by the medical profession has shortened and wasted the "antibiotic age."

A patient, who came into the office with giant urticaria, or hives, taught Dr. McKenna another very important lesson about parenteral vs. oral administration of drugs. These giant hives were dramatic in that they could appear and disappear momentarily and were as big as the palm of your hand. They were recurring of a period of time and became so debilitating that he had to admit the patient to the hospital for treatment with intravenous Benadryl. The constant drip of this antihistamine completely controlled the eruptions. It was dramatic. The logical conclusion would be that when the patient was discharged, with oral Benadryl, the hives would likewise be controlled. Not so. They recurred and were temporarily controlled with intramuscular Benadryl until the use of hypnosis finally afforded a permanent cure. The hives were a stress reaction and parenteral drug administration was far superior to the oral route.

The unorthodox way in which Malcolm's mind worked led him down a lonely road in the overtly rule-ridden group mentality known as the medical profession. Patients came before everything and everybody and political correctness was non-existent. His choice of hobbies was also solitary. He loved farming and fly fishing on the remote upper McKenzie River of his youth.

Chapter XX

Fun Fishing

Malcolm grew up near the Willamette River in Eugene. He enjoyed a "Tom Sawyer" life on the water. He explored, swam, caught frogs and fished. He and his friend, George, built a raft and crossed the wide river to explore no man's land on the other side, an amazing fete of engineering and perseverance for two ten year old kids. He was barefoot from one school year to the next and carried the proverbial bamboo pole over his shoulder.

He became a self-made botanist, entomologist and chemist during his early teens. His bedroom window sill was adorned with bottles containing cocoons and bugs of all descriptions. His mother, out of respect and fear, never touched these things that were so precious to him. A trunk in his closet was covered with oil cloth to create a make shift table and serve as a chemistry lab. He spent hours studying his collection when not in school or enjoying the great outdoors, hunting and fishing.

The McKenzie River, east of Eugene, was a fly fisherman's dream, with its rough white water, swirling eddies and quiet gentle riffles. He taught himself how to fly fish and how to tie perfect fishing flies. Over the years he became an expert boater as well.

The McKenzie was clear, cold and excitingly fast moving. To drift boat there required a special skill. He loved the challenge of it, and when on the river he never ceased to be amazed by its power and its serenity. In later years he would write a poem about his McKenzie.

THE RIVER

How many droplets the river holds
As it flows toward the sea.
Will the same ones return again
In that time called eventually?

I am inspired by the endless flow.
If only I could master such persistence
I would be a revered beacon
To guide those I love through all resistance.

I imagine such strength of purpose
To mold earth and stubborn rock.
Powerful and endless energy to emulate
And become leader of their flock.

It has been said that to be a good fisherman you must think like a fish. To be a good fly fisherman you must also think like a bug. Malcolm's power of observation and application in this sport foretold his exceptional ability as a physician. In those years he had no thoughts about his future. Being totally absorbed in outsmarting the wily rainbow trout was his main focus in life.

The flies that he tied were called beetle bugs. They were split-winged and made of white deer hair, designed to protect the deer from rain water. It has natural oils, is hollow, and very buoyant so that his creations floated well, even in the turbulent waters of the McKenzie. There was no real bug that was called a beetle bug. It was not only designed to float but the white upright wings were easily seen in the glare of day and the darkness of the evening. One must see the fly at all times because when a fish takes it, the hook must be set instantly. Fish don't like the taste of artificial flies and spit them out. This fact adds to the thrill of dry flying. You always see the fish strike, sometimes he'll jump a foot out of the water. The suspense of watching the fly float provocatively is reward enough but when a large colorful rainbow trout smacks it, your pulse races and skillful, tight line retrieval begins. The fish is in his element and uses the current, rocks and downed limbs to his advantage. If you're wading, you move downstream, slipping, sliding and splashing. Oh, what fun! The hunter and gatherer instinct prevails here as it seldom does in our civilized world. These carefree early years deeply imprinted his very soul and he never lost his love of the outdoors.

His fishing prowess came into play during Malcolm's senior year in medical school. A rumor had spread around campus that he was an expert fly fisherman. Ken Mac Donald, who was a bait fisherman, hoped to put Malcolm on the spot.

"Hey, Malcolm, I understand you're a fly fisherman."

"That's right."

"I'm getting together a few guys to go on a trip, over to the Deschutes. Want to come?"

Never one to turn down a chance to fish, he responded, "I'm interested, who's going?"

"Bill Waters and Ed Graham makes up the foursome. We'll shoot for the first weekend in May, okay with you?"

"Count me in."

On the trip to Eastern Oregon, Ken goaded Malcolm. "It's really cold weather this spring. I'm guessing your flies won't be of much interest to the fish. I can loan you some of my salmon eggs."

"Keep your smelly eggs, Ken. I only use dry flies," Malcolm easily returned his needling.

"What if they don't look up? There won't be any bug hatches this early."

"I don't care much, Ken, I just like to float a fly. I'm not a meat fisherman anyway."

"Don't say I didn't offer," Ken said, feeling pretty sure of himself. "How about we each put up five bucks and then give a trophy for the biggest fish?"

Ken thought he was making a safe bet because the lunkers stayed neared the bottom and loved eggs. He knew that fly fisherman always caught the small fish in the shallows. This weekend, as cool as it was, he thought Malcolm was sure to come up empty. He'd be begging for some of his bait before the weekend was over.

Ken drove to the spot he had fished many times, a remote section with giant rocks and deep holes. They set up camp and erected their tent. They had a folding camp table and a two burner stove. It was obvious Ken was an experienced camper and fisherman.

It was about 1:00 p.m. when they hiked down the canyon to the river. The fish weren't biting and after dunking their baits for a few hours, Ken and Ed gave up and headed back to camp.

"Hey, Malcolm, why don't you give up, they aren't even taking eggs."

Malcolm ignored him and moved along, casting his fly on the quiet water. Bill followed him for another half hour before calling it quits. "Malcolm, you are the most optimistic fisherman I ever met. It's too cold out here. I'm heading back for the campfire and a beer." He started to leave, turned back to him and added, "How about you, haven't you had enough yet?"

Malcolm continued up river, "It'll be dark in another hour, I might as well stick it out 'til then. I'll see you in camp."

Malcolm knew that the water he had been fishing was not good for the fly. He also knew that if the fish would feed on top, the best time was just before dark. Shortly after Bill parted, he rounded a bend and was surprised to see a beautiful stretch of shallow riffles. Ideal fly water. Before long a feeding frenzy began. He hooked a trout with every cast. He limited out at fifteen. The largest fish was 18 inches long. His basket was heavy as he walked down the canyon in the darkness.

Ken looked up, beer in hand as Malcolm approached. "I'll give you one thing, Malcolm, you're not a quitter. I suppose you waited 'til we left to charm the fish with your fly," he laughed a smug laugh.

Malcolm opened his basket with the 18-incher on top. "I caught a few."

Ken rose in disbelief. He was speechless. Finally he managed, "Well, I'll be damned. I've never seen anything like this. I always thought bait was the killer."

Malcolm won the trophy, and the respect of his doubting classmates.

Malcolm's fly fishing expertise was demonstrated earlier when he was in pre-med at the U of O in Eugene. Bob Bartlett was an older, married man and an experienced dry fly enthusiast. He had come from Portland to Eugene to go fishing with the kid he had heard was a fly fishing prodigy. Bob's dad worked on the railroad with Malcolm's dad. He strongly suspected Malcolm's dad had exaggerated and was telling tall tales, as proud father's often do.

Bob visited the McKennas that July night before the planned trip up the McKenzie. Malcolm told him that in the hot weather, the lower river was too low and they should fish the upper waters, about sixty miles east of town.

"My wife and I have been looking forward to this, we will enjoy a ride up the McKenzie. We'll pick you up early, what time is best?" He fully expected Malcolm to say something like 4 a.m.

"The fishing is best on the upper river starting about 11:00 to 11:30 a.m. so let's say 9:00 a.m., okay?"

"That's great, we'll be here." Bob admired the water along the McKenzie River Highway and commented frequently. Malcolm countered, "Wait 'til you see the upper river. You can fish there all day without seeing a soul."

The abrupt transition, when they turned off the paved highway onto a dirt road, surprised Bob. The narrow opening led them through giant old growth cedars, tall and majestic.

They arrived at mile post four at 10:30. Bob, who thought that floating a delicate fly on calm water, with room for long back casts, was the way it was always done, was dumbfounded. "You have to be kidding. Are you telling me that anyone can float a fly in this white water?"

Malcolm smiled, "There are plenty of still runs behind the big rocks. The reason that this place is so loaded with fish is that most people are scared off before they try. Here…" Malcolm showed him a handful of his special flies, "…I'll give you some beetle bugs, they float anywhere."

"Now I see why you fish here alone so often. How do you back cast with all that brush?"

"You just roll it out with a flip of your wrist, like this…….. Those flies I gave you will float without a back cast for drying."

"If you say so…." Bob was in no way a believer……yet.

Malcolm was eager and set up long before Bob. "I'll fish downstream and you can go up where it's easier to cast." He left Bob and his wife, Mary, still in a state of disbelief.

It was a calm, warm morning. The air was full of caddis flies, bouncing onto and off the water. "It's going to be a perfect day for this," he anticipated, as he stepped into the cold water. Even with rubber boots and heavy wool socks he felt the chill. He always carried a folding cup in his pocket and now he drank from the unadulterated isolated river. He stood motionless for a while to enjoy the silence and familiar smell of this place so dear to him.

He spotted a caddis riding high on the long, narrow slick that formed behind a moss covered rock in the middle of the river. About half way down to the faster moving tail off, a bright rainbow leaped into the air and onto the fluttering bait. He instantly started a roll of line upstream. When he calculated it was the right length to cross the thirty feet of fast water between him and the prize, he flipped it to his left. He created an arc of line upstream and placed his beetle bug a foot below the rock. It floated directly downstream, high and dry, just as that caddis had done. The rainbow rose, high in the air, with that beetle bug on his nose. When Malcolm set the hook, his rod bent double. The fish darted in all directions, shaking his head to dislodge the fly. He gave it line when it lunged away and retrieved line when it changed direction. The heavy current added to the weight of the 1 ½ pound beauty. It felt lead heavy. This was the adrenalin charged moment he always yearned for. He was ecstatic and fulfilled.

He felt his way downstream, slowly, and repeated that same scene over and over again until his basket felt heavy. He counted fourteen fish, one shy of a legal limit. At that point he hit the road and walked upstream to find Bob and Mary. He was happy knowing they must be near their limit too. He wanted to impress his out of town guests. He did that very thing, but not the way he had expected. He saw Bob sitting on a log near the river below him, and he shouted above the roar of the rushing water, "Great day for fishing, right?"

Bob appeared to be sightseeing and not fishing when Malcolm slid down the hill to him. "How many do you have, Bob?"

"Are you kidding? I can't find one place to float a fly in this raging waterfall," he gestured to the cascading flow before him. "It sure is beautiful, though, and I can see why you like it here so much. How are you doing?"

Malcolm hesitated, "I'm almost afraid to tell you now, but I only need one more to limit out."

"Go to Hell.......You're pulling my leg."

"What about that spot right below you there? Close to the bank….. did you get one there?"

"I don't even see what you're seeing, Malcolm, show me."

Malcolm stepped below him and cast into the fast moving current. Wham! Another 14 inch rainbow! Bob was incredulous. "I obviously can't read this kind of water but you certainly can. I'm mightily impressed, sir." It was getting late when they started back but still enough evening light filled the sky to illuminate the scenic drive home.

"Malcolm, I've fished with some experts, but none the equal of you. I think you really do think like a fish. You should write a book about fly fishing and be sure to put in a chapter on roll casting the dry fly. I watched you, but I just flat out couldn't do it. I was helpless in that break." He added, "I'm serious here, I'll buy the first copy."

* * *

Jill Martin, early on, learned of Malcolm's love of the outdoors and fly fishing. A mountain was their first love rendezvous. He took her camping, often, where they could be alone and away from spying eyes. On one occasion they were sleeping under the stars, by a lake near Mt. Hood, when noises in the night frightened Jill. She always thought that bears were going to eat them. It turned out that they were on a deer trail, by accident, and the deer were bounding over them all night in the darkness. He laughed and tried to reassure her with his homily, "You should fear two legged animals much more than the four legged ones, Jill."

She was intrigued with fly fishing. It looked so graceful and challenging to her. He taught her all the little tricks he had learned throughout his many years of practice and it gave him another excuse to put his arms around her. At those times he found it very difficult to keep his attention on fishing. She was very serious about it, as she was about everything she put her mind to learning. She was always a quick study and soon became as enthusiastic about the sport as he was and almost as skilled.

She was much more patient, however, and would stay put in one spot on the river until she wore down the trout's resistance. Malcolm, on the other hand, was always on the go, using his pent up nervous energy and giving the fish only a few perfect floats to make up their minds.

Finally he announced, "Now you're good enough for a float trip on the McKenzie."

"You mean Canada?" Jill asked with surprise.

"No, there's a McKenzie near Eugene, where I grew up. Wait 'til you see and feel it."

A few weeks later he took her in his drift boat, down the McKenzie. She was thrilled to share this part of his life, this sport he loved so passionately.

They were all alone in his world, drifting. He rowed against the current to control the boat so that he faced the rear seat where she was sitting. Today this view took precedence over even the river. She wanted to get a sun tan and was in skimpy shorts and a thin blouse.

"Feel free to take off the top. We're alone now to do what we want."

"Are you sure? I've never thought I would enjoy a nudist camp, but it's so warm out and this is different in a way." After only a moment's hesitation, her blouse came off, followed quickly by her lacy bra. He rowed with renewed vigor and they seemed to become one with the river. He threw out the anchor in one of his favorite secluded spots and dropped the oars. The sounds and smells of the river and the wide open blue sky above made this sweet interlude nothing less than perfect.

Jill was shocked at how much easier it was to float a fly from the boat. She loved to see those beautiful fish leap from the water so gracefully. It was always a surprise and she had not completely mastered the timing for setting the hook. She did catch a few and was ecstatic. When he pulled the boat into the landing at the end of the day, she hopped out holding the rope for him and looking into his eyes she said simply, "Malcolm, you give me so much joy. I have never been happier in my entire life…..please always love me as much as I love you."

Chapter XXI

Jill and Beth

Malcolm shared two women's love, but a third mistress took up most of his time. Medicine. He was so successful at his practice that he began to feel its lopsided pull. He arranged for another local doctor to trade calls with him. He had been practicing alone now for almost a year. It was very hard for him to think in terms of limits when healing the sick was involved. But he knew he had to, he was running low on "good stress."

Another directional pull was eating on him too. The more he got to know mature and vibrant Jill, the more he realized Beth's child-like tendencies. He went home at night to care for not five, but six children. He would sort out all their individual problems and deal with them, one by one. He had been dealing with patient's problems all day and needed a break. That break only came sporadically when he could be alone with Jill. She was wise enough to acknowledge his needs while subduing her own, to give him the rest he so badly needed. She remained silent about the child she wanted with him and how painful it was for her to share him with another woman. She was always patient and full of joy…..and offered a warm retreat.

Beth must be feeling the pressure of sharing as well. She too remained silent. She could not protect him from all that family pressure and in fact, had become a part of it. What, at first, he thought was an ideal arrangement was showing signs of guilt ridden stress. He did not want to admit, even to himself, that he could not handle the situation he had created. He put it on the back burner. The situation was changing as time passed. Timing was everything.

Two years had gone by since the secret divorce. His children were getting older and more independent. He had been raised a free spirit and thought it had served him well, so he wanted the same for his offspring.

They lived on a small farm which he loved, and by design gave his boys adventure and work. They were never given an allowance but were paid by the hour for doing the chores. A monthly calendar was kept by each. He wanted to teach them two things; a work ethic and the value of a dollar. By the same token, his girls would work in his office when they were twelve, first as chart filers and "go to" help, and then as receptionist fill-ins. He was successful with this approach and none would become smokers or drug dependent; they all became useful, productive citizens.

His major problem was Beth and how to change her dependency issues. He gave it considerable thought. She had not worked outside the home since they were married even though she had bookkeeping skills. Her low self esteem worked against her in any public setting. She loved the seclusion of the farm and giving to her children. She reveled in cleaning, washing clothes and cooking. She ironed everything in sight.

He decided a business she could run would get her out of this agoraphobic rut.

Malcolm had been busy buying up contiguous commercially zoned old houses and lots. This was a continuation of those he purchased along with his clinic building in downtown Stirling. It turned out, in the end, he would own all the property on the block except the part Dr. Welch used to build his clinic on. He also bought two houses across the street from Welch's office; owning a large corner section of the adjacent block. The two-story house on the corner was the oldest house in town. It was unique and in an ideal location for a resale clothing shop for Beth. He visualized how quaint it would be remodeled and applied to city hall for permits.

Dr. Welch used his connections to thwart that plan. Malcolm, at first frustrated, thought about it for a while and then smiled. "So he's still bitter......how sad...but two can play at that game." He chuckled to himself as he thought about letting the old house go to rack and ruin; creating an eyesore for Welch to see every day, out his office window. Renters care less how it looks if the rent is low enough and I save money in the process.

All manner of renters came and went in the old house. A group of young people, to include two comely lassies, occupied it for several years. Gentlemen parked on both sides of the street to visit. Dr. Welch fumed helplessly.

His original plan thwarted, Malcolm rented space on Main Street for

Beth and her shop. It was called "The Cat's Pajamas" and featured upscale resale clothing. This was a popular first in the community. Beth was busy and forced to socialize. The negative cash flow was tax deductible and suited him fine. With Beth so occupied, he could spend a little more time with Jill and not feel guilty about it.

Time was slipping by. It had been five years since his first meeting with Jill at that job interview. It was now three years that he had been living at the farm with Beth and a null and void certificate of marriage in a drawer somewhere. Not one of the town busy bodies knew their secret. Amazing.

Perhaps Jill and Malcolm's relationship was spiced up somewhat when they worked so hard at such a clandestine connection. Jill did have a biological clock problem. She would soon be on the down side of thirty. The temptation for an accidental event was strong but she was too proud for that to be considered. She prayed that he would tire of this double life stress before too much longer. Then again, if he did, in which direction would he turn? She was not sure and it was driving her crazy. She feared Beth's complacency would outlast her patience.

Malcolm had some more pressing problems. The Medical Society was relentless and called him in for "complaints" more frequently. The insurance company's audits showed his billings were higher than the average. This was to be expected, of course, because he did his own x-ray and lab work and made fewer referrals. His fee schedule was the same as others but with the statements not coming from multiple sources, his were higher. The other fact they failed to consider were hospitalizations. His were much lower because his goal was to keep people out of the hospital. Office treatments were much less costly and the patient appreciated being at home.

None of that seemed to matter to those in control who had been influenced by Dr. Welch and friends. He would waste time at those ever escalating evening meetings explaining himself. It was degrading and he resented it, but he had no choice.

"If I ever do make a big mistake, God help me," he foretold, as he left the latest of those crucifixions. "Don't let the bastards beat you down," he remembered from his army days. On his drive back from Portland, he had to smile when he thought about it, realizing what unsatisfactory practices these idiots must have, to think like they did and have so much time to waste. Maybe they were sadists at heart. He lightened up changing his thoughts to Jill; they would leave on a trip in a few days. A week long medical meeting, in Portugal.

* * *

As the plane took off from Portland airport, Jill gripped Malcolm's hand so tightly, it hurt. She was afraid of flying but not so much that she would miss this trip. After takeoff she visibly relaxed and their hand holding was gentle and provocative. She looked at him when he closed his eyes to rest and felt safe and secure. He seemed so in control of every situation, at work or at play. Her love for him was boundless and complete.

They checked into the Ritz Hotel in Lisbon where the meeting was headquartered. It was a marble palace decorated for royalty. "It's so…..so…..Ritzy," she laughed.

"So are you," he countered.

Her height and figure gave the tasteful red dress she wore an elegant air. She was unaware of the effect she had on people, that was part of her charm. Just looking at her made him feel proud.

The doctors at the evening welcome party were captivated. He noticed them noticing her and again was pleased with the knowledge that she belonged only to him.

Dr. Carillo, head of the OB GYN department at the Medical School and president of the Portuguese Medical Society, was instantly at their side introducing himself and ushering them to a front table where he and his wife were seated.

"Isabelle, this is Dr. McKenna and his wife, Jill. They came all the way from Oregon, would you believe?"

Isabelle swallowed hard and fought an instinctive desire to hate the vision in red she was looking at. She was gracious and attentive outwardly. There was much small talk and dinner before the orchestra began to play. Seeing that Dr. McKenna was engrossed in a conversation with Isabelle, Dr. Carillo was quick to stand and invite Jill to dance. He was charming, as most Europeans are, but decidedly more handsome.

She lit up the dance floor, so gallantly displayed by the gregarious Dr. Carillo. Malcolm enjoyed watching Jill from afar. She was usually so close to him that he could not fully appreciate her beauty. When the newly formed couple remained on the dance floor for a quartet of numbers, including a tango, the scene was awe inspiring for the whole crowd of spectators.

"Your husband is quite a dancer, Isabelle, is he always such a good host?"

"He loves people, especially beautiful women and your wife is stunning." Her assumption that they were married stood out in his mind and the idea of Jill as his "wife" was becoming more appealing all the time.

"Would you like to dance?" He stood up to accept her delicate hand. Isabelle reminded him of Beth. She was so quiet and seemed to fade into her surroundings. After two waltzes they returned to their table where Dr. Carillo and Jill were waiting.

"Dr. McKenna, your wife is a magnificent dancer." He had ordered another bottle of the most expensive Portuguese wine and filled the glasses once again. "Here…a toast to Jill, a vision of loveliness from across the sea." They all raised their glasses. With more of the warming beverage, Malcolm, who seldom drank, was feeling relaxed and talkative.

"Dr. Carillo, I'm very interested to know how socialized medicine affects your practice. Is it restricting?"

"Let's not be so formal. I'm Sebastian and you are Malcolm. We are friends now and I intend to be your guide while you are here. I will show you the county hospital tomorrow and everything else you want to see. We can leave here about noon; the meetings will be over then and you have a free afternoon."

"I am overwhelmed by your courtesy, Sebastian, we would love to take you up on that generous offer."

Later, in their room, Malcolm, who was more than a little mellow from the wine and turned on by the sight of Jill, so sought after, pulled her to him as they entered.

"Did I ever tell you how lovely you are? You've been so close to me all these years that I haven't really seen you. Strange how getting away changes ones perspective." She melted into his demanding kiss. Before she fell asleep she thought about her Cinderella evening. She was flattered but mystified by Dr. Carillo, who was so brazenly flirtatious in front of his wife. Most of all she thought about Malcolm. She had never seen him drink quite that much wine. He was so mellow and so happy. She appreciated that he didn't have a jealous bone in his body, but then, why should he? She adored him and he knew it.

Dr. Carillo ushered them through the hotel parking garage to his waiting Mercedes. He drove them to his villa at the edge of town for lunch.

Isabelle was there, with her parents, to greet them. Her parents lived with them which reminded Malcolm of his own home life. Beth's mother had lived with them for over ten years now.

The lunch was dramatically served in courses by their maid. Malcolm was somewhat confused by all this opulence. Dr. Carillo must have been born into wealth or else socialized medicine was not as he had imagined it.

After lunch, Dr. Carillo, leaving Isabelle with her parents, drove them to the hospital for a guided tour. Malcolm was attentive and quick to compare this facility to his. He asked many probing questions.

"How are you paid for your services?"

"Service? I will be frank about this…..if you want service here, you pay under the table." Dr. Carillo's forthrightness surprised Malcolm and explained a lot about socialized medicine and why he prospered in spite of it.

He took them on a tour of Lisbon, pointing out all of its historical landmarks before they picked up Isabelle. The evening he had planned included dinner at his favorite restaurant and then dancing at the Fado. He always managed to seat himself next to Jill. He was so solicitous of her that Malcolm began to feel sorry for Isabelle who looked lonely. Malcolm looked after her and tried to carry on a conversation with her about her past. It was difficult for her to offer more than brief answers. Malcolm had the advantage of understanding her plight because he had dealt with Beth all these years. He was amazed at how much alike Isabelle and Beth were. It was plain to see why Dr. Carillo had been so eager to switch partners. He didn't know, however, just how deep that desire went.

Sebastian ferreted Jill away to the dance floor much of the evening. His small talk was directed to her most of the time. Malcolm did manage to share the conversation sometimes and found Sebastian to be both knowledgeable and likable. He felt the need to have Jill all to himself and made a decision that this would be the end of this foursome. These feelings were justified when Jill talked to him alone in their room later that night.

"I was so uncomfortable. I just didn't know how to handle the situation gracefully. We are in his country and he is such an authority figure. There we were, at that table, his wife and you looking on……and he was exploring my leg with his hand, under cover of the tablecloth. I kept nudging him away but he was persistent. Then on the dance floor he asked if I was happy with you….Can you believe this? He wanted to come over to our room while you are in your meeting tomorrow. I'm still in a state of shock."

"You have to be kidding."

"No, I'm totally serious. I plan to stay close to you…you'll think I'm your shadow. I'll even go to those boring meetings."

"I've never paid much attention to the gossip about European men but I guess I should have," he smiled, "and I have to tell you, I respect your diplomacy in all this. I'm not surprised that he targeted you though, look at you, you're everything any man could want………Did I ever tell you that?" Again the lingering wine and Jill's confession excited him. It was a five star night in a five star hotel………The Ritz, no less.

The next day he told Sebastian that they had other obligations that would fill the remainder of the week. That put an end to the Sebastian Carillo incident.

They would enjoy three free days at the meetings end. Walking near their hotel, they came upon and explored a quaint little art gallery. They were enjoying the many paintings when the curator approached them. "I've been watching you two. Americans, right?"

"How did you know?' Malcolm asked.

"You are such a handsome couple…so open and carefree. You have the western United States written all over you. Am I right?" His smile was friendly and genuine.

"Yes, we are from the west coast. Oregon to be exact, about as far west at it gets," McKenna confirmed, "I'm surprised that you could deduce all that without hearing our accent."

"And you, young lady," he turned toward Jill, "you are classic beauty. You should be on canvas. That would be a shame though, your beauty appears to be multi-dimensional; it comes from the inside out too."

Malcolm thought, "Oh, oh! Here we go again." The short, pudgy, bespectacled little man in front of him did not appear to be the dangerous type, however.

"It's 11:15; almost lunch time. Would you be so kind as to break bread with me in my home? I'm about to leave and close the shop until 4:00 p.m."

They looked at each other in amazement. Was this whole country so friendly? She nodded to him meaning she was game for another adventure. He was feeling the same mystery about this likable little man. "We would love to. By the way, my name is Malcolm and this is Jill."

"I am called Carlos."

The white Citron, parked outside, was better suited to his small stature than theirs but they managed to crowd into the back seat with chins resting on knees. They looked at each other and laughed out loud at the absurdity of it all.

"I see this car is a little cramped for you. I'll bet you're glad we only have sixty miles to go," he laughed too.

"Feels like we're in a phone booth, Carlos, a little tight but the company is great." Malcolm copied his host's humor and seriously hoped he was kidding about the sixty miles. He was, but it was still a fairly long ride out into the country. They were expecting a tiny house, to match his small car and his stature and were astonished when he drove up a winding road to a hilltop sprawling monastery. It was magnificent, standing like a sentinel against the winds of centuries.

"I've been restoring this old place for years," he said proudly. "It's been a long process but I'm very patient." He apologized for its partial disrepair and the towering scaffolding that attested to the restoration under way.

Malcolm and Jill were ushered into a large room with beamed ceilings. Rough cut, well worn hardwood floors led to a massive fireplace that burned invitingly. They sat on heavily carved wooden chairs that were surprisingly comfortable. They faced the fire. Before they could even speak, the butler poured them each a glass of sherry from an ornately charming crystal decanter.

"Alfonso has been with me for most of my life," Carlos said, explaining his presence, "he keeps this fire going. I love to watch the dancing flames, they conjure up all sorts of fantasies….." Carlos went on, "But tell me about yourselves. You young people live in another world so far removed from mine. Please tell all about life in Oregon."

They described the scenic wonders native to their state and then eventually led into some specific Indian lore. Malcolm even told him about his hero, Chief Joseph, and his famous heartfelt speech. "As the sun now stands, I will fight no more forever….."

Carlos was captivated by the enthusiasm and warmth of his foreign guests. He had seen many cowboy and Indian movies; they were his favorites. This made his new friends all the more special. He treated them like royalty and they were served a magnificent seven course lunch by Alfonso.

They toured the monastery and saw walls covered with large tapestries and old paintings. Some were even older than the walls on which they hung. His collection was worth millions. He seemed to be unaware of his wealth, thinking only that these young Americans were the lucky ones.

"If you two are examples of the American west, it must be even more glamorous than I had imagined. You are a perfectly matched set. I salute you," he said with a courtly flourish, "and I wish you long life and much happiness." That was the final toast over glasses of priceless brandy from his cellars. They would never forget this strange little man who had been so generous with his hospitality.

* * *

"Was he a holy man?" Malcolm would ask Jill when something would remind him of that gentle man. "If we returned would that shop and the old monastery really exist? My whole memory of that incident has such a dreamlike quality about it."

"I'm sure he was," Jill's answer was always the same.

That trip to Portugal opened Malcolm's eyes to what his real problem was with Beth. He was so accustomed to her inability to make up her mind and her fear of socializing that he overlooked completely the obvious. He had grown and expanded his horizons. He was thriving on socializing. He always got stuck on the fact that she was so agreeable and he translated that to mean she had no faults. He knew how much she loved him and he felt pangs of guilt when he thought of leaving her. He had truly believed that the two-wife idea would solve his problem. It had worked to the degree that his children were rapidly becoming independent. His eldest daughter had struck out on her own and his eldest son was in the service.

He decided to run a test to see how much he was really needed at home. He closely kept track of how many times his remaining three children would come to him to talk or were in need of him in person. He found himself reading medical journals uninterrupted, for days on end.

He could provide for them, money wise, from a distance and not really be missed.

Beth was like a sixth child. She was always busy elsewhere in the house. She did follow him to bed most of the time. She was very loving in that regard. Her new business was a positive distraction for her but unfortunately she ran the vacuum more at night because of it. After a few months of these mindful observations he decided it was time to make a change.

Jill's son was away at college leaving her with only her teen-aged daughter in her apartment.

"Jill, what would you say if I proposed a change of venue, so to speak?" Malcolm queried. "It really is your turn to put up with me evenings, Beth has done that for over three years now, ever since we started this threesome."

"Do you really mean it?" Jill tried to hide her happiness at that unexpected turn of events.

"I'm afraid so…..nobody really needs me around the farm lately."

Jill wrapped her arms around him. "I need you," she said, "Have you discussed this with Beth?"

"Not yet. I wanted to know how you felt about it first."

"You didn't need to ask. You know I want you with me, anytime, all the time."

Beth was equally surprised to put it mildly. In fact, she was downright shocked at this news.

"I've been painfully aware that people around here don't need me like they used to. I'll be back from time to time to watch over the farm and take care of anything else that has to be attended to," he said gently, "and we'll still have some nights together, if you want."

Beth gave some thought to what she would say next. "I understand what you are saying but I don't like it. I don't want to be left alone here with my mother, you know how she drives me crazy. You are always the referee. You've never said she was a problem."

"And she never has been as far as I'm concerned. I've always liked the tough old gal. She works around here for you, too, that should count for something. Plus she was thoughtful enough to disappear into her room in the evenings when I was home." Malcolm was patiently leading Beth along.

"That's what I mean, if you're not here, she'll be in my hair all day and all night." Beth's throat tightened as she spoke and tears threatened to spill. "I think I'm about to cry…..damn…."

"Come on, Beth, I'll always love you and take care of you," he tried to lighten the moment, "You won't have to feed me or listen to my complaining about the kids. That's the up side."

"I know you'll do what you have your mind set on, regardless. Just remember, you loved me first."

Malcolm knew she would lay a guilt trip on him. He had hoped she would get angry and kick him out. He deserved to suffer over this decision.

He did. Gradualism was definitely not the answer so he bit the bullet and called the family together.

"Kids, I'm very proud of all of you. You're good students and have grown up to be respectable human beings. I take little credit for your accomplishments because I've deliberately raised you up to be independent. Listen up now, carefully, because I will take no credit if you make bad choices and get into trouble either." He looked directly at each young face, "You know the right path and I'll expect you to walk it. Call me whenever you feel the need. I'm going to provide the money for the upkeep here and for your educational needs. And always be respectful of your mother, she deserves that, and she loves you very much. Any questions?"

The silence that followed confirmed his conclusions that he would not be missed and was not needed there. No one seemed surprised by his pronouncement indicating to him that they had been more aware of the situation than he had realized. He hoped that they had understood his parting words. He left the farm for good. He had stayed there four long years after his divorce from Beth.

He hated the confines of apartment living and escaped to the farm acreage to care for the animals and keep an eye on the family. He had been away so much of the time attending to his practice, making house calls and delivering babies that the apartment problem was not insurmountable. He had made his choice and was no longer torn in two directions. Over time he was able to rationalize away the pangs of guilt about Beth. She needed to be free to build a life of her own. One of the town business owners gave her an accounting job when her resale business folded. Naturally, it was one of Dr. Welch's allies who hoped to make trouble for him through Beth.

Chapter XXII

The Promise

Malcolm was living with Jill even though he had promised himself he would never marry again. They had known each other for six years and were very much in love. She wanted a child with him but had never pressed the issue because from early on he had resisted the very idea of ever having more children. A fact he was quite adamant about. Her patience had carried the day thus far against all odds.

That well developed trait even worked for her fly fishing, much to Malcolm's amazement. In later years it would serve her equally well when her artistic ability surfaced. All in all she was an amazing woman and a lot like Malcolm in that she could easily be misunderstood by those who envied her. Their chemistry was based on a deep seated commonality.

Jill's daughter, Paige, from the very beginning, loved Malcolm too. She tried to hide the fact by giving him a hard time. "You're not my father," she would voice many times when he tried to correct her. "But I'm your friend, Paige," was his disarming come back.

In spite of herself, she admired his intelligence and stature as a doctor and there were even times, in the beginning, when she would outright flirt with him. He took it as a compliment.

Paige ultimately found herself in with the wrong crowd in high school. She began wearing rag bag clothes seemingly as a badge of honor. Jill, who was always a fashion statement, found this change in her a hard pill to swallow, and she was having a difficult time communicating with her daughter. She turned to Malcolm for help and welcomed his input.

Malcolm soon tired of Paige's sullenness and so a problem developed between them. He had little tolerance for her behavior and was even more stubborn than Paige herself. The tension soon grew to take on a life of its own and Jill was devastated by it all.

There were times when she feared she would lose Malcolm because of her out of control daughter. Had she had more confidence in his tenacity and ability to solve problems, she would have worried less, but she was too emotionally invested. In the end, he would turn Paige around and perhaps save her life.

They had frequent meetings with the school counselor and with her boyfriend's parents. They visualized Paige taking up with complete strangers and becoming one of those anonymous roadside fatalities.

"This has to stop," Malcolm announced one night, "I feel that she is a danger to herself. She's totally out of control. I thought I could outsmart her, but I can't," he admitted to Jill, after discovering that Paige had sneaked out through her bedroom window to attend a forbidden party.

"I'm frantic, I'm scared to death for her......what can we do?" Jill was crying in his arms.

"I've been thinking about this for awhile and I think we have to send her away to a new environment….a private school somewhere. I hear there are some good ones in Texas and I seem to recall that you had an old girlfriend who lives in Dallas." He looked into her tired face and read the heartache there. "In the morning I want you to call the airline and make a reservation. You need to visit her. You need to get away for a little break and maybe your friend can help you find the kind of school we need."

He knew this plan might kill two birds with one flight. He would be one on one with Paige and with Jill out of the way he would really crack down on her.

Jill welcomed the trip. She renewed her long time friendship with Nita Billings. They had been army wives together in El Paso. Jill's husband had been stationed there when Paige was just a little girl. Even at that tender age she was too friendly and too trusting for her own good. She would walk away with any stranger that talked to her, she thought everybody was her friend. Jill couldn't seem to instill in her a need for caution, ever. Still she never stopped trying.

Jill and Nita found the perfect place for Paige. St. Mary's Academy in San Antonio. There were walls surrounding the school allowing complete isolation and supervision. The student's were chaperoned at all times; their study desks faced the corridor walls for evening homework assignments and lights went out promptly at 10:00 p.m. Weekly trips into town for personal supplies were always in small, well supervised groups. All in all this was a totally structured educational environment, exactly what Paige needed. She called home every weekend and put pressure on her mother.

"Mom, this place is pure Hell," she complained bitterly, "How could you do this to me?" Jill's throat would tighten up with emotion so she couldn't speak and she would hand the phone to Malcolm.

"Paige? We love you……that's why you're there. Buckle down now and study hard, okay? We're very proud of you, you know. You have an opportunity there that most kids would kill for. I know you don't think so now, but someday you'll look back on this and understand. Just hang in there."

At the end of the school year the following June, Paige came home. She was like a different person. She took pride in her dress, she was courteous, and she was respectful in every way. It seemed a miracle had taken place.

Paige would reserve a place deep in her heart for Malcolm. He had saved her from herself and she would always remember. Jill was so relieved and grateful; all was right with this part of her world at last.

"Malcolm, you are always there when I need you," she said appreciatively, "I can't imagine life without you."

Malcolm was thinking ahead to another problem. He was acutely aware of the societal pressure brought to bear on Jill because of their unconventional relationship. He, himself, could care less about society, but he knew it bothered her. It would mean everything to her if her love was validated. She didn't complain, but he knew her so well that when she hurt, he hurt, and conversely, he smiled inside when she was happy.

This was a tug of war for him. He had vowed never to marry again. He weighed his choices. Which was more important? His vow or their vows? He couldn't make a strong enough case for his side.

He awoke early that fateful September Sunday. Jill's body was so warm and so close. He looked at her angelic face; the perfection of it. He thought back on all the fun times they had enjoyed. Her laughter cleansed his soul. With her at his side, he was invincible.

He slipped out of bed, went into the small kitchen and quietly started breakfast. He seldom had the opportunity to cook for her. He was an adventurous chef, a carefree experimenter. Memories of his childhood closet chemistry lab could be relived with dashes of spice. Jill was more conservative but she always tolerated his flights of fancy with good natured diplomacy. She followed the recipes and she was an excellent cook.

He carried a piece of bacon into the bedroom and held it just beneath her nose. Wake up sleeping beauty…..today is special," he crooned.

She came up slowly out of a sound sleep. "Oh, that smells so good."

"And you smell gooder," he said, kissing her cheek. "How would you like breakfast in bed, my little Princess?"

She smiled up at him. "I smell coffee too. Give me a few minutes and I'll meet you in the kitchen."

After breakfast he announced his plans for the day. "How about a drive up the Columbia Gorge? This is going to be one of those spectacular fall days. Can't you feel it? Magic is in the air!"

She knew that when Malcolm used such flowery speech he was up to something. What now, she wondered.

They drove up the old Columbia River highway. Yellow maple leaves were dancing all around on their way to join the blanket of yellow that covered the ground and the roadway ahead. Native dogwoods offered splashes of brilliant red.

"Jill, we are so blessed to have all this right in our own backyard," he said admiringly.

"Oh, look…" she said, "there's Latourelle Falls just ahead, I've always loved it there. Could we stop for just a little while at the falls?"

He answered by pulling into a secluded area that afforded a spectacular view. They sat in the car taking it all in and enjoying the privacy of this location. The very air seemed alive with expectation when Malcolm turned to her and spoke his heart.

"Jill, nature has painted two perfect pictures here. One outside there and one in here beside me." He took her face between his hands and looked deeply into her eyes. "You bedevil me. You haunt me.," his voice filled with emotion, "You make me whole. I love you so much and I want you to marry me. Will you marry me?"

Jill was taken completely by surprise. Her eyes filled with tears. She was speechless, but not for long. "Of course I will…..Of course I will!"

He slipped the ring on her finger and kissed her tenderly and well.

* * *

A medical meeting in Las Vegas was on the docket for December. Malcolm planned a surprise wedding. A close friend, Bill Brant from L.A., would meet them there and be their best man. Bill arrived full of expectation. He and Malcolm were alone in the lobby.

Malcolm was uncomfortable with the message he had to deliver so he just blurted it out unceremoniously. "Bill, I'm sorry, but I changed my mind last night. I just can't do it this way."

"You getting cold feet?" Bill was taken aback.

"Not at all. I just think Jill deserves a big wedding, not an elopement. That rumor mongering small town needs to be hit in the mouth with it. She has suffered their intolerance long enough. I'm glad you're here though. Come on up and meet Jill, but behave yourself, she's mine," he laughed jokingly, "we'll have a good time and have a chance to catch up".

Jill was not told of this close encounter until years later. They made plans for a June wedding.

Chapter XXIII

The Wedding

Malcolm had a flair for surprises and the dramatic. This wedding would be his best effort yet. He was seething inside about Stirling's pettiness and intolerance. Dr. Welch's Marielle and company had taken out their animosity on the guiltless Jill. He was about to shine some light on their treachery and put a stop to it once and for all.

Malcolm knew that Jill was a cosmopolitan girl, but he had to get back to the country. Down deep he had always known the apartment could not be permanent. "Jill, I'm thinking of looking for another little farm, this apartment is stifling me." He watched her closely, not knowing exactly what her reaction would be.

"I'm all for that," she surprised him. She had always known where his heart lay.

"I thought you were city-bred and city-raised, have you been holding back on me?"

Jill laughed. "I guess I never told you about that part of my childhood, did I? I went to grade school in Linton and we lived up Cornelius Pass in a cabin. Jobs were scarce in the thirties and my dad bought some acreage to log. He repaired an old log cabin that was on the property."

Malcolm was fascinated by this new revelation. "Don't stop now, this is getting good," he encouraged her.

"You haven't heard the best part, and you'll love this….we had no running water and the only plumbing was an outside toilet," she said enjoying his reaction.

Disbelief was written across his face. "You're kidding me. I just can't imagine you in that setting."

"I grew up poor, but only in the monetary sense," she went on. "We moved around from house to house in Portland later. My dad would fix them up and sell them for a profit. That's how we survived in those times." He could hear the pride in her voice.

"I know all about that," he countered. "My childhood home near the river in Eugene cost $1,000 in the early thirties. My mother traded her sewing machine in as a down payment and they even had a hard time making the $3.00 a month mortgage. We did have inside plumbing and running water though," he laughed at the memory of it all.

* * *

Malcolm told one of his patients, John Culp, that he wanted some acreage near town. The winter months flew by while they searched. They were getting discouraged because they wanted a place to move into in June, after the wedding.

He spotted an ad in the paper. "40 wooded acres 6 miles east of Sandy. $28,000." That was a little far out, he thought, but they looked at it on the weekend. There was a small, year round stream flowing at the base of a gentle sloping hillside. The timber was dense with no clearing to be found. He discovered that he could drive off Highway 26 and circle above the property. From that upper view, Mt Hood loomed, awesomely near.

"We could do some logging and run a road along the west boundary to the top," he said, bubbling with enthusiastic plans. "What a spot that would be for a house. We'd have an unobstructed view of the mountain and we could build a dam on that stream and have a huge trout pond."

Jill was horrified at this wilderness. It would be full of bears and other wild creatures. "I think we're above the snow line here, we could have deep snow on the road all winter."

"That's a thought," he said, adding happily, "we could get a snowmobile too!"

Malcolm was so excited about the possibilities that Jill remained silent when he called the owner and bought it the next day.

John Culp saved her when he showed them, two months later, a farmstead closer to Sandy. "Doc, wait 'til you see what I've found. It isn't on the market yet. The old German guy, Ed Payne, took it off awhile back. He wanted too much and it didn't sell but I've been able to talk him into a much more realistic price. I just know you'll fall in love with this place."

He continued, his enthusiasm driving his need to share all that he knew about it. "It was homesteaded by the Gibbons family in the mid-eighteen hundreds. They came in a covered wagon from Missouri. A part of the Barlow Trail runs through a corner of it and the actual ruts are still visible if you know where to look.

Payne bought it from them fifty years ago and built the existing stone cottage and barn. Wait 'til you see it." He had hardly bothered to take a breath during his entire narration. John Culp had always talked a hundred miles a minute but now even faster because of his excitement.

He drove through a gate, just off Ten Eyck Road, near Roslyn Lake. They wound down hill through old growth fir trees, past a quaint white barn and stopped at the cottage.

Everywhere Jill looked she saw old world charm. She was relieved to find that this setting was downright urban compared to the alternative. She silently prayed that he would like it too and subdue his Daniel Boone instincts.

They toured the house and barn and then walked down to the small spring fed pond that lay surrounded by cedars. A small flock of grazing sheep kept the grass trimmed so that the setting was park-like.

"What do you think, Doc? Was I right?" John broke the silence.

"I'm overwhelmed, John. If Jill feels like I do at this moment, we'll take it."

Jill put her arms around him in approval. "I hoped you would say that."

They took possession of the farm they would call "Glen Oak" a few weeks later, in April. Malcolm immediately commandeered an old friend, John Roberts, to help him remodel the cottage to Jill's satisfaction.

Time was a factor as the wedding was set for June 26th. Jill agreed to an outside ceremony down by the picturesque pond. There would be no time for a honeymoon in June and they would celebrate by moving from the apartment into the cottage immediately following the big day.

Jill was ecstatic planning all the details. Malcolm was far too busy to interfere and left the "nest building" up to her. The town was abuzz.

"How can he marry her? He's still married," Marielle told her town messenger pigeons. She had hated Jill from the day of that interview six years earlier. She had nicknamed her the "Black Panther" and had predicted that Jill and her then-husband, Jake, were secretly planning to get a big settlement from Dr. McKenna for alienation of affection. Her wishful thinking helped lead the Welch camp down a blind alley.

This wedding, as Malcolm had planned, was going to clear out the town gossip smog with a blast of fresh air. More than a few ladies in town were caught off guard.

"I didn't know he was available," was oft times whispered about now. Most of that town gossip got back to Dr. McKenna through Ben Dobson, who had built the small private Stirling General Hospital. They shared a common theme. The city fathers had always fought his efforts too for some unknown reason. It could have had something to do with the fact that Ben had married a much older rich widow. Her husband had been one of the old timers in Stirling. Even Dr. McKenna suspected the money was the most important to Ben but it was none of his affair. Outsider status made Dr. McKenna and Ben confidants.

The hospital, of course, was ablaze with the wedding talk. The personnel regarded him with deep respect. He had earned their affection with his easy going manner and sense of humor.

Ben wanted to impress Dr. McKenna with a unique wedding gift so he hired a twelve piece string orchestra to play out there among the trees. It was the perfect touch.

* * *

Enter Dr. William Campbell. He and Malcolm were lab partners in pre-med down in Eugene. They planned on sharing living quarters in med school. That idea had been thwarted when Malcolm decided to marry Beth. Instead, Bill served as their best man when they eloped to Vancouver, Washington, just across the river. They were lab partners again, in med school and would always remain friends.

Dr. McKenna had been practicing alone in Stirling, about four years, when Bill visited his office one day. "Malcolm, your waiting room full of patients, tells me that you could use some help here. What do you say?"

Malcolm eagerly agreed. "Let's have lunch and talk it over. I'm free today if that works for you."

They did and Dr. Campbell was a comforting addition to McKenna's overflowing clinic. Dr. Campbell was easy going and the girl's accepted him happily. They were pleased that he would take some pressure off their workaholic boss. It was only natural that Bill would serve as his best man for a second time.

The weather in Oregon can be iffy in June. Betsy Clark, the head nurse at the hospital, was talking about that fact to Dr. Campbell a couple of weeks before the wedding. "I'm really concerned about rain for the big event. I hear Mr. Dobson is supplying an orchestra even. What a shame if we should have a downpour."

Bill laughed out loud at the preposterousness of that suggestion. "It wouldn't dare rain on Malcolm," was his reply. He had observed Malcolm's aura with disbelief for many years. Betsy agreed, hopefully.

She had been one of Dr. McKenna's biggest fans since that day he walked down the hall with her so many years before. "Betsy, you are such a lovely girl. You have tremendous ability and such an easy way with people, I find those qualities really admirable. I have a hard time, though, trying to understand why you would want to mask all that under the odor of cigarettes. It's a little distracting, somehow, were you aware of that?"

Betsy, who was fastidious and knew she was very attractive was stunned by such a remark but took it for what it was worth and immediately put an end to her habit of many years.

She seated herself next to Malcolm in the hospital coffee shop a few months later. "Dr. McKenna, I owe you a debt of gratitude."

"What for, Betsy?

"I haven't had a cigarette since that day we walked down the hall from surgery. Do you recall what you said to me?"

Malcolm knew full well that his carefully chosen words would put Betsy in a double bind situation. He had anticipated the result. "Yes I do and I'm happy for you Betsy.....you do smell good now." They laughed together.

It was a wet June that year. Not heavy downpour, just cloudy, cold, misty wet with an occasional shower thrown in. The 26th, a Saturday, was rapidly approaching. Jill was nearing panic but held back her ever growing anxiety from Malcolm.

"I have all the loose ends tied up and the invitations went out last week. Mrs. Langley has asked to set up a saw horse table in the garage and I thought we could cover it with my grandmother's old checkered tablecloth. It has a lot of sentimental value for me," Jill rambled on happily. "Mrs. Langley and her daughter plan to cook it all in our kitchen and keep that table full of her favorite specialties. The menu sounds spectacular. She's such a wonderful cook and I'm looking forward to something really inspired. I'm sure we won't be disappointed."

Malcolm listened dutifully as Jill ran through the litany of details. He was once again impressed with Jill's ability to tend to minutiae. "Be sure and tell her again how much I appreciate all that effort. She was one of my first patients in the old office," he added reminiscently.

"My sister-in-law's folks are here from Australia," she continued. "You always did admire Sue's accent, remember? Well, hers is tame compared to theirs. Australia is sheep country, at least the part where they come from, so Sue's dad, Jack, loves the idea of a farm wedding. He has volunteered to spruce up the place on Saturday morning. He said something about a 'sheep turd dustpan', whatever that is." She laughed, "Well, at least that's what he called it."

"Sounds like it's coming together. I'm sorry I have to be at the office until noon, but I'd probably just be in the way." He teased, "The cold feet thing you know."

"I'll overlook the cold feet comment if you'll do something about this weather," she said, "I'm getting worried."

"That's all taken care of," he reassured her. "I have an old Indian friend dancing the "no rain" dance this week."

Miraculously on Saturday morning, the clouds parted and a warm sun dried out the landscape. The town was not too surprised and attributed it to Dr. McKenna's hypnotic powers.

Malcolm's friend, Father Bogarth, had retired to the Episcopal Monastery in Sandy where he and Jill visited him a few weeks before the wedding.

"It's been a long time Father. I was surprised to learn that you ended up here in Sandy, our farm is only three miles north." It felt good to see his old friend again. "I came to ask a favor."

Father Bogarth leaned forward, "I'm listening."

"Could you perform the marriage ceremony for us at our farm on June 26th?"

"Dr. McKenna, you have done a lot of good things throughout the years for the church of which only I am aware. I'd be most honored to perform the ceremony for the two of you."

"I'm remiss here," Malcolm stood and gestured toward Jill. "I think this is the first time you've met Jill. She's has been my office nurse for six years and ……"

Father Bogarth interrupted, "Hello, Jill," he smiled at her and extended his hand, "I've heard all about you, believe it or not. You two are quite notorious in Stirling." He turned his attention back to Malcolm. "I've also followed your run-ins with the Medical Society, Dr. McKenna. What a travesty!" He cleared his throat and leaned forward conspiratorially, eager to share guarded secrets. "You may not be aware that you have a powerful friend on the State Medical Board. He has been a strong advocate for you there. He has kept those unprincipled County Society wolves at bay. And there's more...I know all about Dr. Welch's past in all this too. You really stirred up a hornet's nest."

"Tell me something I don't know," Malcolm interrupted, shifting his weight in his chair.

Father Bogarth smiled. "I've even had a few good laughs at how you've outmaneuvered that Stirling bunch. You are undoubtedly aware that they planned to run you out of town?"

A feeling of serenity pervaded the room as Father Bogarth was finally able to expose this long-held truth, this conspiracy. "I was part of Stirling way back before Dr. Welch started out. I know some well-kept secrets."

McKenna was captivated with these revelations.

"The original 'group of 5', as we called them back then, committed many unspeakable acts, including arson for insurance money. They had a very hush-hush sex-club that involved local high school girls and Dr. Welch was a part of that." Stunned silence gave him the opportunity to continue uninterrupted. "One of the group was suspected of poisoning his older wife...he had a younger woman waiting in the wings. That's all ancient history now...you have prevailed over the best influence-peddlers in the business and I salute your courage and your tenacity. Malcolm...you are a *good* man," he added, with an extra emphasis on the word 'good.'

"Father, I'm truly amazed at all this. Thanks for warning me and you've filled in a lot of blank spaces." He rose and offered his hand but Father Bogarth surprised him with a warm embrace that solidified their unique friendship. "God be with you, my son."

Malcolm and Jill walked away from this meeting totally stunned by the numerous revelations so generously offered.

Malcolm spoke first, "Isn't it interesting that friends you didn't know you had, do the most for you?"

Jill smiled knowingly, "Someone is watching over you, Malcolm."

"I was told my Uncle Ray made that very same comment when I was just a baby."

Chapter XXIV

The Big Day

On that magic June 26th the air was electric and clean as only it can be after a month of Oregon rain. The sun was shining through the giant firs with July intensity creating rays of sparkling light on the pond below. The orchestra played soft music that filtered upward and slowly evaporated around the stone cottage.

Malcolm's son, James, and Jill's son, Peter, had volunteered to park the cars in the freshly mowed field near the front entry gate. People walked down the winding road. It was like entering the Land of Oz. 'Surreal' would best describe it. A row of contented cows lined the fence near the barn, seemingly hypnotized by the haunting sounds of violins and cellos. From their enclosure, doves competed with their own soft melody. All the guests were directed to follow the carefully attended grass-covered road to the pond area….the same road which the bride would later travel.

Malcolm and his best man, Bill Campbell, stood on a small plateau of grass at the edge of the pond. The wedding was twice blessed because two robed holy men stood with them. Father Bogarth, in his black monk's robe had brought along Father Eldridge, who was in white. He was the active minister of a nearby Episcopal church. Malcolm did not realize the significance of this until he thought about it later. A monk is not licensed to sign a marriage certificate. The fact that Father Bogarth agreed to attend and did not use that ready-made excuse, told Malcolm what a friend he really was.

The crowd appeared small when compared to the limitless natural surroundings of tall trees. The formally attired musicians were to the left of the crowd where they could see the bride as she began her descent toward her waiting groom. At last "Here Comes the Bride" penetrated the silence.

Jill, dressed in pale green chiffon, was ushered down a grassy trail by Elizabeth, Malcolm's sister. It was a long circuitous route compensating for the steepness of the hill, adding to the bride's dramatic approach. It seemed an eternity that Malcolm watched and waited. His knees trembled and his throat was parched.

He hardly heard what the robed holy men said, but he somehow regrounded and placed the ring on Jill's finger at the appropriate moment. He repeated the vows, "With this ring I thee wed……..to have and to hold……..from this day forward….." She placed a matching band on his finger and squeezed his hand. It was her turn. "To love and to honor…… from this day forward……."

They were married at last. People watched the sentimental touch of the planting of a young oak sapling where they had stood together just moments before. The coup de gras came when they propped a large bronze plaque at its base. It read: *This oak stands where Jill Martin and Malcolm McKenna became man and wife. June 26, 1971.*

The McKenna crest also adorned the plaque with crossed sword and oak tree. It would later be permanently imbedded in a huge boulder base where it remains to this day beside the oak tree, a sixty foot monument to their union.

The crowd drifted slowly up the hill to the cottage to enjoy Mrs. Langley's food and champagne. The festivities spilled over into the late evening. Jill and Malcolm slept blissfully in their new bedroom that night. All was right with their world.

That summer and fall at Glen Oak was peaceful and energizing for both Jill and Malcolm. He arose at 5 a.m. one Sunday morning; climbed the ladder to the hay loft and stood in its open doorway high up under the peak of the barn roof. He looked out over his pasture and woodlands. He shouted out for all the world to hear, "I have a beautiful wife and a beautiful farm. I'm the luckiest man alive!"

Grim reality would set in a few weeks later, unfortunately.

The first New Year's Eve after their June wedding turned out to be a tale of two families. Malcolm thought the plans were well made for two of his children to spend some vacation time with two of Jill's children. It didn't work out that way and not only did it put a strain on the newlyweds but it would leave the two camps even more alienated.

It all started innocently enough when a patient suggested, in September, that Dr. McKenna use his condo in Sun Valley for the holidays. The owners were going to be in Europe instead. Malcolm polled his five children and it turned out that one daughter, Jean, and one son, Sean wanted to go. A promise was made. Jill's daughter was in Texas and her son was in Eugene attending college. At that early date they had no plans to come home.

"It will give you some one on one time with Jean and Sean," Malcolm said, knowing this was a rare opportunity for these three to become better acquainted. "We'll have a good time. They will be off doing their own thing as young people always are, and while they're off, I'll teach you how to ice skate," he offered gallantly, realizing his own lack of expertise would lead to some memorable moments. "You always said you wanted to learn, right?"

"I've never been to Sun Valley," she smiled at him. The thought of it excited her, "It sounds perfect for the holidays. I just wish Paige and Peter were coming too though." Then at the last minute Jill's children had a change of heart and wanted to be home for Christmas but would have to leave early before New Year's.

Jill was torn. "I can't refuse to spend Christmas with my kids. What can I do?"

Malcolm was disappointed by this turn of events but put on a happy face.

"Why don't you fly over on December 30th ? That way at least we can have New Year's together," he offered as a compromise. "Don't feel bad about this, we'll have a lifetime of Christmases together, this can't be helped," he tried to be cheerful. "I already have the tickets and my kids have planned this for months. I can't change it now."

When all was said and done, the new plan sounded like a perfect solution and Malcolm, Sean and Jean left for Sun Valley, as planned, on December 21st. Jill hosted Paige and Peter at the farm. The newlyweds had to spend their first Christmas apart but their sacrifice would keep everybody else happy. They had not counted on the snow storm that moved in on Christmas Eve, perfect timing for a white Christmas.

It turned out to be bad timing for the Sun Valley plans though because snow piled up and they were snowed in at the farm for a full week. Jill missed New Year's with Malcolm and she missed the whole Sun Valley experience. She did enjoy her one on one time with her family but that was a hard one for the new bride to forget.

Malcolm's oldest daughter, Jean, was very close to him and was having some problems with the marriage anyway. She couldn't help but see Jill as an intruder. Jill had hoped the trip would help that situation but it only made it worse. His daughter had him to herself for the holidays and she made the most of it.

Chapter XXV

The New Arrival In Town

Malcolm's previous farm experience consisted solely of raising beef cattle. He inherited a small flock of twelve sheep with Glen Oak. The story is always told about cattlemen's hatred of sheep. Sheep graze the pastures much shorter than cattle and they eat anything, including Tansy Ragwort, which is poisonous to cows and horses. He took a page out of previous owner, Ed Payne's book and kept the sheep in the back pasture around the pond to maintain the park-like setting. Cattle were heavy footed and would muddy up the pond. Their droppings were not as aesthetic as those little firm pellets left by the sheep, for sure.

He found the sheep much easier to control. If you could get one to go into the coral, they all followed, one by one, in a line. Jill much preferred them because of their size and temperament.

The big steers, even when they were just coming into the barn to get hay, scared her. She thought they were chasing her, when in truth they were just curious. Nevertheless, she always armed herself with a big heavy stick, just in case.

Cows seem to know when you fear them and always want to get closer as a friendly gesture. They would rub their heads against Jill's stick.

There was one black-horned steer that she named "Billy Sunday". He was wild-eyed and a jumper. He could jump any fence and he did frequently. One rainy night in October, they were awakened by a terrible commotion near their bedroom window. Billy Sunday had jumped not one, but three fences and was in with the sheep. He had his horns caught in their feeder which was a sawed off old hot water tank. It was heavy galvanized metal. The sound of horns on metal and metal on rocks was deafening in the middle of the peaceful quietness of the country at night. Jill held a lantern while Malcolm pried him loose with a long crowbar. It was more than a little dangerous and definitely frustrating. Billy Sunday ended up locked in the barn and was sold within the week.

"Maybe we should switch over exclusively to sheep," she suggested, when they got into the shower covered with mud and blood. A horn had broken off during the ruckus and blood was everywhere.

"I was thinking rabbits might be an even better idea," Malcolm laughed.

Clashing horns awoke them on a few other occasions. Buck deer would fight near their bedroom windows. Jill didn't complain but she was fearful of the solid blackness outside. There were no close neighbors and no city lights to keep her company. She was afraid for Malcolm when he would take walks alone at night to check things out. She thought he must be part owl and foolishly brave.

"Aren't you afraid out there?" she questioned, looking for reassurance.

"Afraid of what?" he would admonish her. "It's too dark for most two-legged animals, and as I've told you before, those are the only kind you need to fear."

Their admiration for sheep was tested in the spring when it was shearing time. It always looked so easy and Malcolm was eager to try out the electric shears that Ed Payne had left behind. They dawned coveralls and went at it one Sunday. Jill put on her best brave face and was very pleased with herself as she helped by holding the round wooly bodies in an upright sitting position.

Malcolm's knowledge of anatomy worked in his favor. He made very few skin cuts. After a couple of sheep he realized how strong a shearer had to be. His back and arms were killing him, but they kept at it until evening and finally corralled the last one.

"We should have started with this one," he jested, trying to straighten up once again.

"I think we should hire a professional shearer next time," was Jill's opinion. They smelled like wet wool and were oily with lanolin when they headed for the shower. He hugged her tightly, "You're such a good sport. I love you anyway, even if you do smell like ewe." She had to laugh, as tired as she was. "Never lose that sense of humor," she punched him playfully, "It always keeps me going."

That first summer, when the fields were dotted with bales of hay, Malcolm had a plan. He thought about Earl Weinstein, the college president. Wouldn't he and those college professors look out of place hauling hay to the barn? He really admired Earl and that feeling was mutual so it was natural that they loved to tease each other with one-upmanship ideas.

Following a board meeting at the college, he cornered the president. "Earl, I have 400 bales in the field that need to be stacked upstairs in the barn. Could you and a few of your professor muscle men help me out? We'll have a keg party afterwards to celebrate."

"Great idea, Doc, how about this coming Sunday?" Earl knew he would have as much fun challenging some of his staff as Malcolm did putting him on the spot.

Shaking hands to seal the bargain, Malcolm said with eager anticipation, "It's a go then. I'll get the beer and set up some poles so we can catch trout to barbeque. The pond is loaded with twelve-inchers right now."

The hay party was even more fun than Malcolm had anticipated. The out of shape crew of five professors and their overweight president were like fish out of water. Much sweat and tears of laughter later, they somehow got the job done.

Malcolm did his share and then some. His muscles were more accustomed to farm labors. The unbelievable part was the fishing. After hitting the keg too hard his elite crew couldn't hook a single fish, so Malcolm had to step in and save the day. He had drunk only the cold spring water. They feasted that night on fresh trout and corn from his prolific garden. Dr. Weinstein teased that in no way could Dr. McKenna maintain a weedless, perfect garden like that by himself.

Jill defended him, "You are kidding, I hope, he's outside in it until dark almost every night."

That unconventional party was a huge success and the talk of the campus in the weeks to follow. Those that missed it felt slighted.

* * *

Jill and Malcolm had been on the farm well over a year when he drove her to the Chanticleer restaurant in Portland, one evening, after closing the office. "We need to celebrate tonight. You've been working those cattle pretty hard lately," he teased.

"You make fun of me but I did help with the shearing and the lambing despite all those awful sheep ticks. I love those little helpless lambs though."

She grimaced and added, "But the cows are something else, I think cows are for cowboys."

They sat at the same table downstairs that they had many years ago when they were in hiding. "I want to make a toast," he said, holding his glass high, "This is to the baby."

"The baby? What baby?" Jill was at a loss.

"The baby we're going to have," he announced smugly, "and it will be a girl!"

"This is crazy talk….I'm not even pregnant and," she was becoming intrigued with this conversation, "how would you know it would be a girl?"

"It's up to me on both counts. I rest my case," he said confidently.

Jill's heart was racing at the thought of a baby. She was now thirty seven and borderline too old to think of such a thing anymore. "You always have delighted in shocking me but this tops it all." Her eyes glistened with tears of pure joy. "Are you sure you want a baby? You've said so many times that you didn't."

"I said I'd never get married again too," he grinned. "Now you're making a liar out of me twice over."

She reached across the table and took his warm hand in hers. "I pray your deeds can match your words. Now what about that girl, what will she be like, I wonder. Will she have your penchant for figures…and I do mean math figures here…and my love of the arts?"

"That would be the fine arts, I presume," he countered glibly, "and not the two handsome Arts that come into the office."

"You can joke all you want, but is the world ready for such a woman?" she wondered. "Your brass and my class, a deadly combination for sure."

* * *

The wait was not long. Three months later a very excited Jill was pregnant.

"She'll be delivered by her father, on the farm, with hypnosis," Malcolm proudly proclaimed upon hearing the news.

That got Jill's attention. "Wait a minute now, I might have something to say about that. I want to be in the hospital. Remember I told you how I hemorrhaged with Paige?"

"That was the Army for you. You're in good hands now, and there will be no bleeding." His confidence did not completely satisfy Jill. She was older and had to worry about Mongolism too. But she would put the delivery out of her mind for now.

"I've planted a good seed," he boasted. "This baby girl will be healthy and beautiful, just like you."

Her due date was January 29th, which was rapidly approaching as the months flew by. It was an icy night in December when their car blew a water pump and overheated on a steep hill a few blocks from home. They walked gingerly on the icy road. He held her arm with a protective grip.

"Oh, look at that full moon, it's so bright out here tonight." She slowly turned around to enjoy the view in every direction and squeezed his hand tightly. "We're so lucky to be right here at this very moment."

"Jill, you're such a good sport." He smiled and made a point of glancing down at her very large belly. "You're almost as big as that full moon, too."

"I am not…and to prove it I'll race you to the gate."

"Like Hell you will….steady now, one step at a time."

Jill grew rapidly from that point on. She could not get up from the rug when they would lie down in front of the fireplace to watch TV. January came and went.

"I was due ten days ago, do you think something is wrong?" she asked worriedly.

Malcolm reassured her, "Not at all. The due date is manmade and your body will tell you the exact time. I think maybe it takes a little longer to create perfection," he smiled.

Malcolm kept a sterile delivery kit handy at the farm knowing it should be anytime now. He did not plan on traveling to the hospital in the middle of the night. He had to reassure Jill on a daily and sometimes hourly basis. She felt like a manatee on land. Each day that passed added to her fears and discomfort. As usual, Malcolm had a plan that he did not share with Jill. By this time she desperately wanted a C-Section for instant relief.

He knew they were only days away from February 14th. A girl would, all her life, be blessed with Valentine's Day to celebrate her birthday. He thought it was predestined. A day at a time he waited with anticipation to that end. Jill's anticipation was not in sync with his.

February 14th arrived at long last. "Jill, I'm taking you to the hospital on my way to the office this morning," he announced at breakfast.

"Whatever for? I haven't had a hint of any labor yet."

"You will have. Our baby girl is going to be born today. It's Valentine's Day."

"Oh, why didn't I think of that?" she said mockingly. "It's too perfect!"

Jill thought about her dreamer husband all the way to town. Most of the time she thought she knew him but this was insane. He took her to the hospital admitting desk and wrote orders which included buccal pit, a little pill that dissolves in the mouth and when absorbed gives a very minimal and safe stimulation to the uterine muscles. He went across the street to the office where his schedule looked hectic at best.

At noon he ran over to the OB wing. Jill was up walking the hall. He felt her glare when he opened the swinging doors. "I'm still here, what now?" She had lost her sense of humor.

"Be patient," he reassured. "I promise you, today is the day, and I would like you to have our baby between 5:00 and 7:00p.m., if you can manage it. The office is booked solid to 5:00 and I have a College Board meeting at 8:00. Would you concentrate on that, please?" He was dead serious.

"Sure," she shot back, "How about 6 o'clock?"

"Great," he said, glad to have that settled. "I'm off to make rounds and then back to the office. I'll see you shortly after 5:00 and I do appreciate your cooperation in this, you're a sweetheart." He kissed her cheek as he turned to run.

Jill watched him as he raced out the door. She wondered at his energy level. She felt so tired and useless right now.

He came back through those same swinging doors about 5:15 as scheduled. She was walking in the hall again, still hoping.

The head OB nurse was just exiting Jill's room and turning the corner into the hallway when Malcolm confronted her with an order. "Fran, let's get her into bed and bring me the sterile kit for membrane rupturing. We'll get this going now." He was all business.

He examined the cervix. It was soft and ready. She was two fingers dilated. He gently punctured the bulging membrane. Fluid gushed out. It was clear, a sign that all was well with the baby. He had heard normal heart tones abdominally before this procedure. He reinforced her hypnosis level.

"I'm going over to the cafeteria for a quick bite. This will be the only chance I have to eat tonight. Call me when she goes into delivery." He ran out the doors only minutes after he had entered. It was 5:35.

He was paged at 5:55 and ran quickly to the dressing room to change. Urgency was repeated from the delivery room. He barely had time for a quick scrub. Through the open doorway he called out, "Hold it, Jill..... Breathe through your mouth." She was already draped. He was hurriedly gowned and gloved. She was crowning when he stood ready to control the birth. He put gentle pressure on the head.

"You can push now……easy…….easy…..control that urge to bear down too hard. Give me a gentle push….there we are……..slowly now. Good job."

The head was out and the perineum was intact, no laceration. He suctioned the fluid from the nose and around the little mouth. "The face and head look like a girl to me," he announced. "How about another easy push?"

It was a girl. She was so pink. Her eyes opened to look at him as if to say, "Where am I, it's cold out here."

"Is she normal?" Despite all his reassurances Jill was still haunted by her nine months of fear.

"She's beautiful and so lively," a big proud smile covered his face. He clamped and cut the cord then showed her off to Jill. "See our beautiful baby girl, special delivery for Valentine's Day. Have you ever had a better present?"

Jill stared for several seconds at her perfectly formed daughter. She was so relieved and thrilled at the same time that she didn't think to call him on his smugness. The nurse held the baby for her to admire while Dr. McKenna delivered the placenta and then massaged the uterus to get it to contract.

"Very good, no bleeding now," he said to no one in particular. He smiled at Jill, "You can relax about blood transfusions, you're all done and you did a fantastic job."

Malcolm had suffered a slight catastrophe though, in his haste to get into the delivery room, he hadn't tied the drawstring on his scrub pants tight enough and they had fallen down around his ankles.

"Nurse, would you mind taking off my pants so I can move?" He smiled, knowing how his request would sound to the new nurse. Her look of complete disbelief said it all.

Malcolm stayed with Jill and their newborn until 7:30 and then ran off to his College Board meeting. When he told them of the exciting event which had taken place less than two hours previously they were flabbergasted. "And you're here? We think you had a good enough excuse to miss this meeting."

"Are you kidding? I have to keep you guys honest," he said in jest. "You'll spend too much of the taxpayer's money if I turn my back for a second."

"You're an amazing man, Doc. No man that I know of would be here under these circumstances. I like your style and I like your wife too. You're one lucky guy." Dr. Weinstein walked out with Dr. McKenna after the meeting.

"I know that, Earl," he acknowledged. "I appreciate your devotion to this college too. You've created a monument to yourself here."

Malcolm returned to the hospital to be with Jill. He sat on the edge of her bed, holding her hand. "Have you counted her fingers and toes yet? She's perfect…..just like you said she would be. Why do I ever doubt you? We've done something really wonderful here, haven't we?"

"We're naming her Gabrielle, right?" He questioned her even though he was still opting for 'Brooke.' In his mind he thought the name Jill had chosen was a little haughty, but he knew he could shorten it to 'Elle.'

"She is Gabrielle Grace," Jill insisted. Another maverick McKenna had arrived in town.

Chapter XXVI

Fertile Fields

Everything written in books is worth much less than the experience of one physician who reflects and reasons.
Rbazes 850-923 A.D.

Surprisingly enough what he learned on the farm would help Dr. McKenna heal the sick. He had grown up watching his father turn the earth, one shovel at a time. Every year in the spring, he would sit on the porch and wonder, "Why does he turn those leaves under so carefully along with all the chicken manure?"

Each year in the fall the city trucks would bring loads of maple leaves that were swept off the tree lined streets.

The garden was large on their city corner lot, occupying almost a fourth of it. He watched it grow and turn those leaves into corn, carrots and potatoes.

He would feed the flock of chickens they raised on the back corner. The chickens lived in a house made of newer boards than the ones that lined his bedroom walls. He gathered eggs often, still warm in his cold little hands. He watched his father butcher fryers and stewers. His love for the soil and what it could produce started there. He later vowed he would raise his children on a farm and not in the city. He did. That decision would prove to be fortuitous in unexpected ways.

* * *

The plants in his garden grew tall and green when fed mineral-rich manure. He knew that people, like those plants, needed proper nutrition and minerals to survive and be healthy. He postulated that most, if not all, disease was due to malnutrition. *Treat the cause and not the symptoms* seemed logical to him.

He frequently dealt with sick animals and became a veterinarian by default. He was amazed at what could be learned about people diseases while treating animal diseases. Some of his apparently healthy calves would die suddenly. It seemed paradoxical to him that the fattest, best looking calves were affected and the scrawny ones survived this strange illness. This could not be an infectious process.

He read that a local veterinary college was doing some research on "White Muscle Disease." In this disease the heart muscle of young animals would be replaced by scar tissue and look white at autopsy. It could be said that this was a form of premature heart attacks and lead to sudden death. This appeared to be a new problem historically speaking. How could it be non-infectious and new?

That riddle was finally solved. It was a mineral deficiency disease. The mineral was selenium. At that time medical doctors thought that rare metals belonged on the atomic table and not on their treatment table. Dr. McKenna gave all of his new born calves an injection of "Bo Se", a combination of selenium and vitamin E, a synergist. He had no more dead calves. From that point on, cattle salt blocks would be available with selenium, as well as iodine. He used them.

Dr. McKenna, the veterinarian, had cured his cattle but he wanted to know why the selenium deficiency had occurred in the first place. Could people have trace mineral disease? His powers of observation would answer that question.

In western Oregon, the heavy spring rains would produce lush pasture grass if you applied ammonium sulfate or urea chemical fertilizer in February. This was standard practice for farmers who were becoming much more educated and efficient than their forebears. A Eureka moment came when Dr. McKenna observed his cows put out on that lush green pasture for the first time in the spring. They congregated along the fence lines, eating weeds and yellowed grass that had not been fertilized before they touched the tall green grass.

"Why?" he puzzled and soon he answered his own question. Sulfur in that fertilizer can be taken up by the plants when selenium is unavailable. They were looking for selenium. Animals are innately able to search for proper nutrition. People can't do that and are vulnerable. "My father was an organic gardener by default because commercial fertilizers were unheard of in those days. We ate mineral-rich produce unknowingly," he thought, "We didn't have a family doctor because we were seldom ill." This new found knowledge added credence to Dr. McKenna's cautious acceptance of drugs which are man-made and chemical in nature. The human body was not made to process unnatural substances. Harmful side effects should be expected.

Treating chemically caused disease with more chemicals didn't make sense. He had always used as few prescriptions as possible and would now write even fewer.

These heart attacks in juvenile cattle treated with Bo-Se sparked his interest in vitamins and minerals. He read all available literature and soon discovered knowledge in this area was sadly lacking.

He became a fan of Dr. Linus Pauling, an Oregon State University professor, who had zeroed in on Vitamin C. Interesting again, to note that OSU was a veterinary and not a medical school.

Dr. Pauling postulated that high doses of Vitamin C would cure viral illnesses. He was a controversial figure in the medical world. Dr. McKenna thought that Dr. Pauling's experiments substantiated the fact that Vitamin C did fortify cellular membranes to prevent viruses from entering. It was well known that viruses must do their damage intracellularly.

Dr. McKenna also thought that Dr. Pauling's idea of mega doses orally was flawed. He felt that blood levels could not be raised by that method. He also knew that those dosages would be excreted in the urine and could cause kidney stones.

Double blind studies by others failed to get the expected results causing medical doctors to doubt the whole concept.

Dr. McKenna called on his experience with his famous hives patient to bring forth an argument for raising blood levels of Vitamin C by giving it parenterally and bypassing the stomach. He found a lab in the Midwest that manufactured vials of Vitamin C for IV administration. The vial was hourglass shaped with two compartments. The unstable Vitamin C crystals at one end and the liquid solvent at the other. When pressure was exerted on the solvent end by way of a movable rubber stopper, a center stopper moved as well and the liquid sterile Vitamin C was produced.

He administered these 10cc dosages intravenously which resulted in an instantaneous high blood level. He gave these shots himself because if any of the weak acid leaked out of the vein it would cause swelling and pain. The nurses were happy to have him usurp this part of their job. It was a nuisance factor for him and used up some of his valuable time.

He did prove his point and began offering a cure for many viral diseases like mononucleosis, hepatitis, and herpes (shingles), these were common problems that could have serious side effects. He was the only doctor in the area offering such a treatment and of course many word of mouth patients came to his clinic. Patients were ecstatic to find help when they had been told there was no treatment available for their problem. No hospitalizations were required for serious complications of these diseases as in the past.

He was saving the insurance companies thousands of dollars and reducing patient suffering. He was a hero to them but their short-sighted insurers complained about the multiple shots.

The Medical Society was quick to agree that this was not standard treatment. The "Shot Doctor" was out of control once again. He informed his patients that their insurance would not pay before he gave these treatments. It was up to them to choose. They usually elected to pay out of their own pockets and were seldom disappointed by the result. Dr. McKenna proved once again to be ahead of his time and was singled out because of it.

His frustration was dwarfed by the frustrations of those politicians who had to deal with this unconventional maverick. Their blue book never did cover what ailed him. He had broken no hard and fast rules. Over time they would spend a lot of money trying to catch him with a breach of ethics.

In spite of them he continued to heal the sick. His reputation spread far and wide. He was a spokesman for proper nutrition long before that word would become common place.

"If man makes it, always beware. If nature makes it, consider it good for you. Eat everything but in small portions," was his mantra.

When serious illness presented itself to him he was quick to recognize it and acted accordingly. Richard Sparks, a long time patient and good friend, came in one afternoon. "Doc, I just don't feel good somehow."

Dr. McKenna began with the usual questions. "Do you have any pain?"

"Not really, but I've lost my appetite."

McKenna knew that Richard was not a complainer. Even though he looked fine at first, he ordered a complete physical.

During the workup the blood chemistry suggested unsuspected liver disease. He thought the liver's edge felt slightly irregular also. To shorten a long story, liver cancer was the diagnosis.

"Richard, I'll be very honest with you. There is definitely no good treatment for this. If I send you to an oncologist they will put something together. What they do will make you feel much worse than you do now. If I were in your shoes, I'd do whatever would make me happy while I still felt able. I'd do all those things that we tend to put off 'til later. In your case it is later."

"How long do I have, Doc?"

"I can't tell you that for sure but less than one year is a good guess," was his honest answer. "I don't usually suggest this but your case is well suited, and you're a good friend. We could try hypnotherapy. Your own immune system can cure anything given a chance. No side effects for sure."

"Let me think about this, Doc. I'll talk it over with my wife and daughter."

He did that and as Dr. McKenna anticipated, they wanted a referral to the oncologist. He would never have made a case for hypnosis had he not felt so close to Richard. Well meaning relatives always go for treatment, even bad treatment. It's human nature not to give up. They had no way of knowing that hypnotherapy, in Dr. McKenna's hands, could be the only chance for cure in this case. He could not guarantee anything, but he felt strongly that Richard's own T cells enhanced through hypnosis, was the best bet here.

The oncologist suggested surgical biopsy to better define the cancer. Dr. McKenna complied, going against his strong feelings that this was a bad decision. Surgery was performed and a biopsy taken before chemotherapy was prescribed.

This surgery forced Richard, who was feeling well at this time, to cancel a golf tournament he had long been looking forward to. He didn't attend and he didn't leave the hospital. A deadly reaction to the treatment ended all his plans.

Dr. McKenna foresaw this result. He was devastated that his friend was gone within two months of the unexpected diagnosis of liver cancer. He knew that the mind was capable of increasing T cells and curing cancer but he would never have the chance to prove it. Organized medicine would continue on their path of cutting it out and killing it with chemicals. He knew that we would look back someday and be appalled at that illogical method.

Dr. McKenna approached healing using prevention and nutrition with renewed vigor. The problem with this unconventional approach was obvious. How could you ever prove what you had prevented?

Chapter XXVII

The Conspiracy Surfaces

The mystery man that Father Bogarth had told Dr. McKenna about finally retired from the State Medical Board. The man who had protected him for many years was gone. With that buffer lifted, the dirty work started so many years before by Dr. Welch and company resurfaced. At the time all malpractice insurance for the State of Oregon was issued under direct control of that Board.

An official letter was sent to Dr. McKenna in April. "After a complete review of your file, we are sorry to report that your malpractice insurance must be cancelled as of June 1st."

Dr. McKenna, who had never had a malpractice claim, was perplexed but not too surprised. He ignored that warning and continued his practice without coverage. A brave move that astounded the perpetrators.

They stepped up their harassment with more notices to appear at the County Society offices in Portland, mostly to answer insurance company complaints. His patients were not a party to all this and, in fact, were completely unaware of his plight.

He practiced for four years without insurance and with continual absurd special treatment by the Medical Society. They wasted his time and tried his patience until he decided enough was enough. He contacted Tom Brewster, a Portland attorney, who had become notorious for winning malpractice cases against Oregon doctors.

"What you've told me is incredible," was Mr. Brewster's initial reaction. "This is a classical case of conspiracy, I've never seen such a persistent effort," he shook his head in disbelief. "This Dr. Welch really hates your guts. He has done everything except hire a hit man. You must have done a lot of things right to deserve such attention." He stood offering McKenna his hand, "I will take your case on contingency. I have worked against those people long enough to be aware of how little they know about due process."

"Thanks, counselor, I hope we can end all this once and for all." McKenna left Brewster's office feeling somewhat refreshed and empowered.

A lawsuit was promptly filed against the Oregon Medical Society to include the county society as well. A doctor suing his own societies was unheard of and surprised everyone involved.

A month later, Dr. McKenna met with Tom Brewster in his Portland office. He was smiling. "Doc, you have no idea what these zealots have been up to. I saw your file. It's six inches thick. They have even hired shills to go into your office disguised as patients. They have scrutinized your billings of Medicare and insurance companies. They were looking for fraud. They spent thousands of dollars and came up empty……no wonder they hate you so much."

McKenna smiled knowingly, "I'm not surprised. What do we do now?"

"Well, we have a problem I hadn't anticipated. You have an iron clad case except for one small detail. Damages. Because you stopped paying insurance premiums and were not sued, they actually saved you money. They have not been the cause of any mental breakdown or loss of income or treatment costs. We have no monetary damages and unfortunately at this time in Oregon, you cannot sue for mental anguish."

McKenna was incredulous, "You mean we have to drop the case?"

"We do, but they will reinstate your insurance, without question. I appreciate this opportunity you have given me to look inside those offices. It's even worse than I thought, but maybe they'll lay off you for a while now."

That lawsuit did quiet things on the medical political front, but the small town cadre of gossipers and city government Welch people was persistent.

Dr. McKenna had always been interested in real estate as evidenced by his original clinic construction and later buy- out.

His original farm, on the edge of town, could have been serviced by a branch of the sewer line that was under consideration. That line would have extended to a high school where sewage was being pumped and hauled, at considerable expense to taxpayers. It was pure malice and short sightedness that influenced the city council to vote it down….their reason being that it would have made Dr. McKenna's property much more valuable.

Another such vote with Dr. McKenna in mind, negated development of an additional sixty-five acres that he owned bordering a main road with sewer in place. These votes blocked the logical extension of the city boundary to the east. The taxpayers were once again damaged because that sewer line would be underutilized and the tax base would have been greatly enlarged with houses that were not built.

The owners of the clothing store, who had hired Beth, were hard at work to further the cause. They offered her an attorney so that she could take Dr. McKenna to court for more alimony support. She was not so easily influenced as they had hoped. She told him everything. He had always maintained close contact with her and helped her and the family when they needed him.

That same store owner had some college connections and attempted to sabotage his influence there. Dr. Weinstein would laugh and tell him of her efforts. "Doc, these people are vicious. What did you do to them?"

"I survived, Earl………I survived."

He went on to become board chairman in spite of their efforts. He always worked hard to help build a strong college and protect the taxpayers.

It may have provided Dr. Welch, et.al., with busy work all those years but their fruitless destructive efforts had little effect on Malcolm. His practice flourished.

* * *

Ben Dobson was desperate for a doctor to cover his emergency room. There were no ER physicians in those days. He was talking to his friend, Malcolm one afternoon. "Doc, your office is across the street. Could we work out some deal for you to cover the ER during your office hours?"

"I'm really booked up solid, Ben, but I would like to help you out." He thought a moment, "I'll tell you what.…if you send all ambulatory patients over to the office, we'll work them in. I will run across the street to take care of the serious injuries."

Ben was relieved. "You have a deal, Doc. I do appreciate it."

That handshake agreement, between friends, set up an amazing chain reaction. Dr. McKenna loved "good" stress and it was a good thing. He would run across the street and admit patients. If they had no family doctor he wrote orders and followed up with whatever care was needed. For every patient he went over to see, two or three came across the other way. His office surgery and x-ray could handle every minor emergency patient.

In addition to caring for his regular patients, he was sewing up lacerations and putting on casts everyday.

On one occasion, four ambulances pulled into the ER lot. Eight patients from an auto accident up the mountain were brought in to the hospital. He had the head nurse at his side with charts as he gave each one a cursory exam. She wrote orders and routed them to the surgery or x-ray or to the floor for admission.

Fortunately, it was near the end of the day and his office cancelled only four patients. One by one he sutured, casted fractures or kept them for observation. He worked for three hours into the evening but by then each had received his full attention and was properly cared for. The nurses, who were running in all directions, were duly impressed. He loved his work. He arrived home for dinner at nine.

"That must have been some accident. Sit down…you look tired." Jill was so understanding because she knew exactly what his work entailed.

"That chili sure smells good, I'm so hungry, I feel like I could eat a horse. I'll have two bowls with onions on top."

He crashed on the couch soon after, she covered him gently with a blanket and slid a pillow beneath his head.

Chapter XXVIII

His Call To The Wild

Malcolm was an avid bow hunter. He loved the sport because he could enjoy the outdoors in the same way the Indians had in the past.

"Jill, bow hunting season starts in a few weeks. Would you like to play Indian with me?" he asked, hoping she would be as enthusiastic about this adventure as he was.

"I'd love to go. I can't pull a bow but I'd like to watch."

"I'll make reservations at a horse camp I know up in the Wallowas. Wait 'til you see Eagle Cap," he said, excitement mounting in his voice. "We can ride a trail almost to the top. They call that country little Switzerland."

Jill was thrilled at the prospect, they hadn't had a break in awhile. "I can hardly wait. You definitely need to get away for a rest."

He reserved a cabin at the camp aptly named *End of the Road*. The accommodations were rustic but quaint. The wood cook stove and the outhouse reminded Jill of her childhood on Cornelius Pass. They arrived about 4:00 in the afternoon.

"Let's break out the fly rods. Listen," he said shushing her, "that's the Little Minum River you hear over there. It flows down from Eagle Cap." Jill could hear the excitement beginning to build in his voice. "We'll be following it up to its birth place in the morning."

"The air smells so good up here," she said, rummaging through her creel, "what fly should I use?" Jill felt the rush of excitement too, as she put her pole together.

They caught a dozen six-inch trout for dinner. "The fish are small up here but wait 'til you taste them," he said savoring the memory of past feats. "Fry them crisp and you can eat them bones and all," he took the spatula from her. "Here, let me help you with that."

"I'm making sheep-herder potatoes too," Jill was already peeling the onions to go in them. "This reminds me of that cabin up at Mt. Hood. Do you remember?"

"Are you kidding? My life began there." He wrapped his arms around her waist. "We'll christen this one the same way, if you're up to it," he grinned.

"Now you are kidding. I brought this bottle of champagne in anticipation of a repeat performance!"

They were up at 5:00 eating pancakes, eggs and bacon. "What an appetite you have, mighty hunter…." She piled the ready pancakes onto a serving plate. "I have a couple more cakes here…" she offered.

"I'll take 'em. We have a big day ahead, wait 'til you see that big buck I'm going to get. We'll eat venison liver tonight," he promised.

"I brought a whole sack of onions. I'm prepared."

He held a jacket ready, "Put on this sheep skin coat. It's really cold up here 'til noon. You will never guess it's August. There will be patches of snow where we're going too," he cautioned.

The horses were saddled and waiting when they walked over to the corral. Neither of them had been on a horse in years and it felt strange as they started up the trail. The smell and sounds of the horses snorting billows of steam into the frosty air added to the excitement and anticipation.

"We should get out like this more often, I can see already why you love to hunt. The beauty of this pristine wilderness almost takes my breath away." When she could take her eyes off the panorama before her, she turned to him, "Your horse's name is Homer, right? Strange name, don't you think? I like mine better, she's called Ginger," she said, patting her mare on the neck.

"You sure do talk a lot up here. At home I don't hear a peep out of you for an hour or two this early. When we get up the trail a ways, we'll have to be quiet. We are hunting, you know." Malcolm held his bow with arrow at the ready.

The trail ascended the mountain through large broken granite rocks. Alpine firs survived here and there. It was like a planted rock garden. The clicking of the horse's shoes on the graveled granite was musical.

"Oh look," Jill pointed, whispering, "there's one now."

"I saw it when we rounded that turn back there," he whispered back, "it's a doe. I don't shoot the ladies. They're too beautiful."

"That doesn't seem fair somehow. I'll bet those bucks with their huge antlers are just as beautiful, maybe even more so."

"It's fair," he said emphatically. "The bucks know how to hide and one buck has a harem of does. They need to be thinned out, otherwise they kill each other fighting over the females. Just like men."

Jill interrupted to cut short this line of convoluted logic. She could see where he was headed. "I don't think so. That's wishful thinking. No harem for you."

They reached the trail's end about 1:00 p.m. He helped Jill off Ginger. They spread a blanket in a grassy clearing and ate their lunch. They drank from the cold river that was only a foot-wide at this elevation.

"See the snow over there?" he said gesturing. "We're really in the high country here."

Jill stretched a little, "My stiff muscles tell me we've ridden a long way. How far did we come?"

"About eight miles. It was in this very spot that I camped years ago. Dr. Huntington and his son and I brought my oldest son too. In fact, if you followed that deer trail over there, you would find the spot where James shot his first deer with his bow. I'm sure he'll never forget that."

"Is that the same Dr. Huntington we've had out to the farm for dinner? You two have been friends for a really long time, haven't you?"

"That's the one. I've known Rich since I started private practice. He's a hell of a surgeon. We've operated together ever since then, that's how I got to know him so well. He flies a plane, did you know that? We flew all the way to Mexico for marlin fishing more than once."

"How could you do that? Small planes really scare me."

"I want to take you marlin fishing in Mexico. You'd love it. We'll take a commercial flight though," he reassured her.

They finally headed back down the trail with their coats tied down behind the saddles. It was warm now. Several does crossed their paths but no bucks until they were close to camp. The horses plodded going up, but liked to trot coming home. They smelled the promise of oats. In any event, they were in a hurry now.

There, on his right, stood two four point bucks about twenty feet off the trail. He drew back his arrow slowly and aimed at the front shoulder of the lead buck. Then, just as he was about to release the shot, Homer became impatient and took off for home.

"Whoa! Whoa, damn it!" With his hands busy, Malcolm could not pull back on the reins. His careful aim was shattered as his arrow fell off the nock.

"You miserable nag," he muttered under his breath, "I'm going to kill you when we get back!"

Jill who was following down the trail burst out in loud laughter. "That was a real Kodak moment. I sure wish I had had a camera. You should have seen yourself………It was priceless!"

Malcolm wanted to cry. "I didn't think it was so damn funny," he said, not finding any humor in the situation yet. But he recovered quickly with, "No deer liver for you tonight, smarty."

When they dismounted, after the long hours in the saddle, they found their legs seemed permanently bowed. They could barely walk. In the cabin they spent the first hour fighting cramping leg muscles. When that passed, the next obstacle presented itself. They couldn't sit, they piled their bed pillows on the kitchen chairs and tried again. No better. They looked at each other and suddenly were hysterical with laughter.

"You should have had my view of that," she said, holding her sides to keep them from hurting as the scene flashed before her once more.

"I know. I'll bet it was funny to you. You don't realize that Chief Joseph is turning in his grave because a stupid horse destroyed my image. But I think I've solved one mystery. Now I know why they called my horse Homer. That's all he was good for…….. going home."

Some moments are indelible.

* * *

Two years later, Malcolm made good on his promise and planned a trip to Cabo San Lucas, marlin fishing. They flew to La Paz and then drove a rental car all the way down to the tip of the Baja peninsula. In those days the road was not well developed. They visited remote Mexican villages and watched wild donkeys with cactus needles embedded in their noses, run along the roadside. Laborers with broad straw hats, pushing old wheelbarrows were repairing the roadway at times.

"This is so exciting! I feel like we're explorers." Jill broke the silence of the long drive.

"We're in pretty primitive country here. Not a good place for a flat tire or worse," he observed. "This is a new car though, only 5,281 miles on it," he read from the odometer. "I guess we'll be okay."

"I wonder how Cabo San Lucas ended up in such a remote location?"

"It's a fishing village. I think the tuna and marlin like the warmer water farther south."

"I can't wait to see it," Jill said, anxiously.

Cabo was a sleepy village on the shore of the sea of Cortez. The buildings were mostly tin-roofed houses. They drove into the parking lot of the only hotel. It was a one story building that wedged itself into the rocks of the sloping shore line. The lobby was a happy place with mariachi music playing.

The bellhop came to them as they entered with two, fishbowl sized margaritas in hand.

"I'll trade these for your luggage," the young man said, handing one to each of them. "Here you are. You can register right over there. My name is Pedro if you need me."

The quaint hotel oozed hospitality and ambiance. The sea air flowed through windowless arches.

"Malcolm, this place is so unexpected and perfect, can you believe it?"

"I think that parched long drive sets you up. You can't help but be impressed and relax here."

Their room was equally as charming. The windows were louvered with no glass so that fresh air was everywhere. It was getting late and they were famished. After a quick shower, they headed for the dining room, Jill's dark hair and carefully selected floral dress made her seem a native. She was gorgeous as usual. No one could resist staring at this handsome couple as they entered. They thoroughly enjoyed the meal of authentic local dishes. Just before dessert sounds of muted trumpets approached the dining room from far down the beach. As it drew nearer they recognized the beautiful melodious strains of *Spanish Eyes*.

A young woman, dressed in a sequined gown, rose unexpectedly from her table and began to sing. Her voice was exquisite. It was so spontaneous they wondered if it was part of the planned entertainment, but they were told later that she was just another guest. It seemed like a scene straight from a musical, so appropriate for this carefree evening. Everyone stood and clapped in appreciation when she finished.

Malcolm moved his chair closer to Jill's and put his arm around her shoulders. He was moved by the event they had just shared. He kissed her cheek softly.

"Malcolm, you are such a romantic. I admire everything you do, but at times like this I'm especially touched. People never get to see the real you as I do," she said, taking his hand in hers. "I love you."

A simple, "I love you more," spoke volumes in return.

The sea was calm the next day except for a few rolling, low profile swells. Unfortunately, that was all it took for Jill to get seasick. She was lying down below the whole time and didn't get to see Malcolm land a 200-pound marlin. She couldn't take the action shots of the event that he had wanted. They did have some pictures of the two of them on land with his huge fish hanging between them, for a souvenir.

They spent the remainder of the trip exploring the isolated beaches nearby. It was amazing that they could be all alone on miles of beautiful white sand with exploding waves for a sound track, and never see another soul. He took some risque footage of Jill cavorting nude there. He brought his 16-mm professional camera that he had picked up in Hollywood from a friend, years earlier. It had come with many lenses and filters and he wanted to try them all out on his captive model. The camera liked her.

It was a trip to remember and they arrived home refreshed and eager for the challenges that lay ahead.

Chapter XXIX

The Time Factor

Drs. Walters and McKenna had practiced together for about ten years when they were joined by Dr. Edelson. He had been the ER physician at the hospital across the street for almost three years. Tiring of that, he decided to try private practice and approached Dr. McKenna. "I have been amazed by the sheer volume of cars going in and out of your parking lot. It looks like you could use some help. I think you're aware of how impressed I am with your approach to the practice of medicine. ER patients give me the opportunity to compare local doctors and you certainly rose to the top of my list." He took a deep breath and added hopefully, "I'd like to be your third associate."

"I'm flattered Don, I have observed your practice too. You impress me in that you are genuinely concerned about the patients. Let me talk to Dr. Walters about it. The building is set up to accommodate three easily."

When Dr. Edelson joined the group a few months later, Dr. McKenna had more time off to pursue his many diverse interests. The first thing he did was to increase his hypnosis practice. Time had always been a limitation that he resented and he knew he could expand this method in many directions. He made greater use of *age regression*, more challenging and more productive for the most difficult cases. By now, he was very comfortable with this method.

Fran Foster was a perfect candidate. She was an attractive twenty-five year old who had suffered from severe headaches since childhood. She had seen innumerable doctors over the years and had had a complete work up by a Portland neurologist a few months before she saw Dr. McKenna.

"Doctor, I'm probably wasting your time," she apologized. "Everyone says its nerves."

"From your history I would agree that there is no organic illness here but the waste basket term "nerves" covers a lot of territory. You are a good candidate for hypnosis." He was thinking ahead about age regression as a quick method to discover the cause of her headaches. They had been a problem since about age twelve and he knew that a childhood incident must be involved.

After three sessions he was getting her down deep enough to try. "You are on a train. It is stopped at the station. See the sign out the window? It reads Thursday 1978. The train begins to back up....faster and faster now....1977....1976....1975," he droned on, his voice growing soothing and softer. "You will watch out that window until you see the date and the incident that started your headaches. When you arrive there, tell me what you see."

In a child's voice she began, "I'm sitting on a couch next to my grandfather. He is smoking a cigar. It smells so bad. My mother is bringing my birthday cake with candles. I blow out the candles. I cough."

"How many candles?"

"Four."

Now that he had uncovered the secret that even she was unaware of, he began the return journey to the present. "I'm bringing you back now.... the train moves forward.... you are looking out the windows....you see the signs....the train will stop at the station and the sign reads 1978....you will be rested and refreshed, just as though you had had a full night's sleep. You can wake up now."

On further questioning, Dr. McKenna discovered that when Fran was four her mother and father divorced, she moved to Spokane and they lived with her grandparents for a few years then. The divorce and move was the traumatic incident and smoke could be the trigger.

"When you get headaches, do you smell smoke?"

Momentarily she was perplexed by his question and then it dawned on her that smoke was always involved. "That's right," she said excitedly, "I do, and if I'm in a smoky room I always get the headache."

Dr. McKenna put her back down, there in Spokane, at the next session. He erased the trigger. Fran never had another headache. He repeated this scenario, with minor variations, many times.

He had another interesting block of patients....children with learning disabilities. Young people are the best subjects for hypnosis. Their minds see everything literally and are not yet clouded by forced knowledge. He could remove mental blocks that led to reading, writing, or mathematical under achievement. He always yearned for a chance to start with a whole class of five-year-olds and use mass hypnosis. He ventured a guess that they would excel in all basic skills when compared to any other routinely taught group.

Word of his successful treatment, with hypnosis, spread. He was sought after to give talks at colleges and fraternal organizations. To add a touch of class and drama he would be flanked at the head table by two tall beauties, Hillary and Jill. He preconditioned them to respond to a single word induction with an instant deep trance. He incorporated that word in his talk at an appropriate time and one of the two girls would instantly close her eyes and totally relax into a visible trance state. A few moments later the other girl would likewise respond. Totally unexpected, this created a dramatic and memorable example of the hypnotic trance. He would then hold up one of their hands and put a needle through it. He, in that manner, demonstrated pain control and also control of bleeding when the needle was removed and no blood appeared. He told them that he was placing an ice cube on the back of their extended hand and, sure enough, a cube-shaped blanched area would appear in spite of the fact that he had no ice.

Word induction was safe, he thought, because only his voice could be accepted. He always removed that word's power when he brought them up out of the trance. On one occasion, however, he slipped up. Jill had been induced with the word *nurse*. Later in the afternoon, on the same day as the luncheon demonstration, Jill was assisting him in the office surgery. She was standing at the supply counter getting some sutures when he accidentally used the word *nurse* while talking to the patient. He waited for the suture and then looked over to see her in a trance, leaning against the counter. They laughed about that incident many times but he never forgot to remove the induction word again.

Malcolm was a voracious reader and catalogued in his mind tidbits of unrelated information. He had complete recall and would put these facts together at an appropriate time. He had more time to read now that the clinic was so well staffed. One piece of historical information that had been so remembered was the story of a French doctor who had written an article near the end of World War 1. That doctor had observed that soldiers who suffered poison gas burns healed leaving unblemished flawless skin. It was as though the old skin had been peeled off and new almost baby-like skin grew to take its place. Microscopically he noted that the hair follicles dipped inward and were not burned. These areas served to seed the new growth.

Another medical article appeared later describing how another French MD had resurrected the original treatise and did research using various chemicals similar to mustard gas to do what he called chemical peels, at first on pigs and finally on humans. His perfected formula was secret but had recently been used by visiting MDs. Dr. Stein was one such doctor who practiced in Florida. Dr. McKenna contacted him and eventually went to his clinic for first hand instruction. He was stunned when he saw some of his patients. They were women in their fifties and sixties who appeared twenty years younger. Their fine facial wrinkles and other sun damage had been totally erased.

Dr. McKenna instantly saw the possibilities. He was once again ahead of his time. This was an era before the plastic surgery craze that would engulf the country. He had been healing the sick all these years and now he could fight aging.

Many of his women patients had psychological illnesses because they feared getting old. He had one patient he recalled who had huge freckles all of her life. She hated them and that hate lead to an inferiority complex. There were scores of acne damaged faces too. Women especially, but some men as well, wanted clear skin like movie stars seemed to have. Dr. McKenna had always treated this problem with reassurance and that tired "beauty is only skin deep" philosophy. He knew that such an approach changed nothing and these people continued to hurt down deep.

He spent three weeks with Dr. Stein and mastered the procedure. Dr. Stein wanted to pass along this secret that he had learned in Paris. Doctors are teachers first, it has been said. Dr. McKenna, back in Stirling, started by giving friends and acquaintances a free face peel. Jill volunteered to be first in line because she had seen and talked to those Florida women. Her result was, as expected, amazing. She talked to new patients about the procedure from then on. The fact that the doctor would do this for his own wife proved that it had to be safe. Her natural beauty enhanced the result, obviously.

Word gradually spread and a local TV station picked up on it. McKenna appeared there with Jill and some other patients. The program deluged his practice with women who wanted to look like Jill. He was very selective and told about half of the prospects that this procedure could not remove deep wrinkles or sagging jaw lines. He referred them for plastic surgery.

* * *

Dr. Cherry was a young, unknown plastic surgeon from Portland who had made an appearance at Stirling General Hospital early on when he was starting out. Most established plastic surgeons would not travel that far. He even became a permanent staff member and attended monthly meetings. Most other specialists were associate-status only and were not required to attend them.

Dr. McKenna first met Dr. Cherry when he had been called in as a consultant on an accident victim with extensive facial lacerations. McKenna closely observed how he treated the surgical nurses. He could see that he was a prima donna in the making and he did not like him from the start. He would not refer patients to him. He knew instinctively why Dr. Cherry traveled so far to be on staff and was so solicitous. Dr. McKenna could also see that Dr. Cherry would have a hard time building a referral practice. Plastic surgery depended on referrals completely. Dr. Cherry served on the medical records committee when Dr. McKenna was Chief of Staff and always reviewed those committee's reports. He saw that Dr. Cherry was absurdly critical with his reviews. McKenna thought to himself that he would likely be another medical society recruit.

Dr. McKenna was polite and civil but that did not hide his mistrust of Dr. Cherry, who resigned from the staff and retreated to the big city within a year. Dr. McKenna was a pioneer in the area of facial peel and Dr. Cherry was the first to feel threatened. He was incensed by McKenna's audacity. This should be a plastic surgery procedure. He would get none of Dr. McKenna's numerous referrals. With his departure from Stirling General, Dr. McKenna buried Dr. Cherry deep in the past.

The ubiquitous Dr. McKenna was busy healing every manner of illness. He made use of conventional medicine along with vitamins, nutrition, hypnosis, and now chemical peels. Nothing escaped his radar. His success was uplifting and he was oblivious to the wolves at his heels.

Chapter XXX

The End of an Era

Caution had always been Dr. McKenna's byword. First of all, do no harm. With the face peel procedure he was alert to the fact that this was strictly elective. He turned many candidates away. He required the patient to fill out a psychological and medical history of previous illness form. He did a cursory physical exam including an electrocardiogram. He always installed an IV tube so that he could administer sedation when needed. The line was also open so that he could give drugs for allergic reaction for cardiac arrhythmia.

He could have sent the patients home after this outpatient procedure but he took one additional step of precaution. He leased a nearby private facility where they would not be seen in public. The face was covered mummy-like in tape. He had a nurse stay there with them as well. They would be discharged in 72 hours, after the tape was removed.

The peel was basically a third degree burn. Such a deep burn on a small portion of the body is of no great consequence. If areas are extensive then fluid loss and electrolyte imbalance can occur. This was not the case here. He was doing peels with an increasing frequency and had soon reached the magic number…100.

He had had no complications because he was so selective with screening procedures. If he felt the patient wanted the peel for the wrong reason, he turned them away. They should only want it to make them feel good about themselves and not to please a mate or someone else. There were limitations as to what problems the peels could correct. He referred some to plastic surgeons if they needed surgical procedures. The patients he selected, however, were getting amazing results. He had a professional photographer take before and after pictures for his records.

Because of these results, patients were walking testimonials and the word spread quickly. He was now doing two or three peels a week. He was becoming concerned this would take over his practice and he didn't want that to happen. He wanted to do all that he was capable of to heal anyone in need. A waiting list became a necessity for the peel procedure.

Dr. McKenna should have been more suspicious when fifty-year old Mrs. Benedict said, "I just want to look like your wife. Her skin is so young and flawless."

He didn't become too alarmed at the remark because every woman he saw wanted to look like Jill. Where he went wrong was not paying enough attention to how she said the first half of that statement. She really expected to be a different person. It was not new skin she wanted. She wanted all her problems solved. She wanted to be Jill. He reread the forms she submitted later, but found no problems there.

Dr. McKenna told her he would like to talk with her husband but she said he was on a business trip in China and would not return for a month. He quizzed her carefully about her diabetic problem. He wanted to get medical records from her family doctor. She cleverly side stepped the issue by stating she took care of it herself and had not seen any doctor recently. These were all red flags that Dr. McKenna missed. He had asked all the right questions. She had falsified the answers. She was a severe diabetic and not borderline as she had claimed. He did do a blood count and blood sugar on her, at the time of the peel. It was normal. She had no blood pressure or arrhythmia problems during the event monitoring.

Then the inevitable happened. She died in a diabetic coma, 24 hours after the peel.

For the first time in his life Dr. McKenna shut down inside. He was heartbroken. He had caused a death. Mr. Benedict came into his office the next day. Dr. McKenna explained. "I'm so sorry. I don't know how this could have happened. I am always so careful to check everything."

"Doctor, I understand all this better than you ever could." Surprisingly Mr. Benedict showed deep sympathy for the distraught doctor. "You were duped. She lied to you. She and I had major marital problems. I don't hold you responsible at all. Every doctor she ever saw was completely frustrated by her. They all talked to me about the problem. She was the most stubborn, controlling woman in the world. She did what she wanted, always…right down to the lie that I was out of the country."

"Mr. Benedict, is there anything I can do for you?" Getting no response, McKenna arose from behind his desk and extended his hand. "I appreciate your honesty."

"No, I'm okay doctor. I apologize for the pain she has put you through."

That should have been the end of the story. It wasn't. A sleeping giant had been awakened. At last the Medical Society held something real to work with.

The charge was "gross negligence." He was advised to get an attorney to represent him in the so called court proceedings that would be held a few weeks hence. He and Jill made an appointment with Tom Brewster, the lawyer who had represented him when he sued the Medical Society many years earlier. The thought was that this attorney knew all about the conspiracy and could therefore best represent him. The problem with this plan was that Mr. Brewster was always after huge contingency fees from doctor's insurance. He did not want to take a case on an hourly fee basis. What he said aloud was, "I'm so booked right now that I couldn't give your case my undivided attention." He referred them to Mark Billings, who was an MD and an attorney.

As they walked to the elevator, Jill could no longer control the feelings that boiled inside. "That was a strange conversation in there. He obviously was aware of what they are trying to do to you and yet he refused to help. Why?"

"Money, Jill," he said tiredly, "with lawyers it's always the money. Justice is blind and never the issue. Lawyers can take either side of a case with impunity as long as they get paid. Whatever lawyer I hire will want a big sum deposited in his office trust account and he will draw from that. Doctors treat first and hope to collect later. That's why I write off about 20% of my charges after spending a huge sum in overhead to collect the rest. If you stop to think about it, doctors are not very good business men. They are so busy curing people that they become sitting ducks for lawyers waiting to pounce. When lawyers make mistakes, they get paid anyway and who is waiting to get them? Not doctors, that's for sure."

"Well this whole thing is not fair. There has never been a more devoted and caring doctor. Every time you get out of bed in the middle of the night, I wonder how you do it. This is your reward for all that?"

"I guess, as they say, my reward will be in heaven, Jill. There is nothing on earth that is fair," he said, bitterness in his voice. "Strike that word *fair* from your vocabulary."

Dr. McKenna blindly followed Mr. Brewster's advice and made an appointment with Mark Billings. The idea of the doctor-lawyer combination sounded ideal to him. He was too busy and too off balance from the charges to ask himself the obvious questions.

What kind of a doctor would become a lawyer? He certainly wouldn't. How would an inexperienced lawyer be able to deal with the complexity of a conspiracy? Later he would conclude that Mark Billings had been a mediocre MD who sought refuge by becoming a mediocre lawyer. He also would realize that Tom Brewster had taken his case so many years before because he wanted a good look at the inner sanctum of medicine to further his own lucrative practice of attacking doctors.

He had never been a friend of Dr. McKenna. Friends are rare and the last place to look for one would be in the legal profession.

His original lawsuit against the Medical Society would have changed everything had it gone to court. It didn't, because of money.

The kangaroo court date was rapidly approaching and Dr. McKenna was puzzled that Mark Billings was not lining up witnesses for his defense. Medical colleagues could verify how proficient he was. Office personnel could speak to Mrs. Benedict's character and subterfuge. Nothing was happening, he thought.

Mark Billings did have a plan. He knew that Dr. McKenna would get no justice in the upcoming hearing. He was going to get the whole process transferred to civil court in Portland.

Dr. McKenna, Jill and Mark sat waiting in the court room of Judge Wilkerson on that fateful Friday afternoon. Three Medical Society attorneys sat smugly nearby. The judge finally appeared.

"I'm sorry gentlemen, but I must excuse myself from this case. Dr. McKenna is my wife's doctor."

Surprised silence flooded the room. The three Society attorneys were thinking…How could this inept, maverick doctor out in Stirling be Portland Judge Wilkerson's family doctor?

Little did these lawyers realize that many Portlanders were traveling the distance to see Dr. McKenna. They were indignant about being forced to come to this court to start with and now were furious that everyone was waiting another hour with no judge.

Finally a new judge was found and called all the lawyers collectively to the bench. Mark Billings returned and said a trial was to take place now. He looked pale and confused. He thought today was to be a trial date setting. He was unprepared for this turn of events. If he had been a more mature lawyer he would have told the judge he needed to have witnesses and be ready, but he didn't.

It was a farce. The Society lawyers lied about the case. The judge was grumpy and in the dark about why he was involved at all. Mark Billings plan was sound but he blew it. They walked out too face a kangaroo court in two weeks.

That hearing consisted of twelve state and county board members and the three attorneys. They were seated on one side of a long table. Jill, Dr. McKenna and Mark Billings were facing them.

It was informal to a fault. Rapid fire questioning with no input from Mark Billings. He had not brought forward a single witness.

They brought Dr. Cherry, the plastic surgeon that Dr. McKenna had rejected so many years ago. To see him there, as part of the Medical Society crucifixion did not surprise Dr. McKenna. He was surprised, however, by the venom of his testimony. He literally nailed Dr. McKenna to the cross.

"Facial peels are in the realm of plastic surgery and should never be done by other MDs. This is a pure and simple case of gross negligence," he said vengefully.

That testimony, completely unanswered by the defense was deadly. Mark Billings had presented a well written answer to the charges. He proved, on paper, that the grounds for gross negligence were not met. If this had been a due process hearing, that was sufficient. There was no due process in this travesty of justice.

Most all the members of that lynch mob had had malpractice suits in the past. One of them had three pending at the time. Dr. McKenna had none.

The maximum penalty was handed down by a unanimous vote. Revocation of Dr. McKenna's license to practice medicine.

Dr. McKenna was not really surprised. He felt victorious in a way because it had taken them thirty-five years to finally have their envy requited. Everyone close to him was totally stunned in disbelief. His colleagues, his patients and his family could not imagine how a doctor with his knowledge and experience could be suddenly cut off from such a successful practice. It was a true tragedy of the greatest magnitude.

The feeling of being martyred helped Malcolm adjust and retire to his farm but down deep inside it was like a cancer eating away at his very soul. He tried hard not to let it show which caused him to become despondent. Jill did not know this man. She only knew the eternal optimist, the man who could move mountains. His sense of humor vanished.

"Malcolm," she pleaded, "please come back to me……I need you."

"What are you saying? I'm right here."

"It's not you standing there, it's a total stranger."

Malcolm was fighting with that stranger too. He wanted him to go away. Jill seemed to him oblivious to his inner turmoil. "How could she not know me after all these years, is she that naïve? Or am I the greatest actor of all time? I've alienated everyone closest to me, including myself." His heart sank. "Where do I go now?"

He would sit out by the barn with Gypsy, his faithful dog. Hours would go by.

"You're the only one who really understands me Gypsy…it's just you and me against the world."

I suppose it was natural under the circumstances that he would grow to trust no human being, even Jill. No one could possibly understand what a toll all those years of making it all happen had taken on this man. He had been so devoted to his patients and his family, actually two families. He felt that he had carried the weight of the whole world on his shoulders.

This was classical depression. He was in a deep dark hole.

"Malcolm, I've made an appointment for you to see Dr. Walters. You need to talk to someone who understands all this, I can't seem to help you……….I don't know how."

"Thanks Jill, but I can work this out. I know I'm my own worst enemy right now but I'm the only one that can fix it."

His resentment toward Jill deepened. She was the one who should be there for him…..not some doctor. He had always been there for her.

His love turned to all the animals. He cared for them with a passion. He understood them. They were not complex and corrupt like humans. Gypsy's love was unconditional and always had been. She would wait on the porch and run to the car each time he returned. She would put her head in his lap when he opened the car door and look up at him, her eyes glazed over with pure adoration and low mournful moaning would fill the air. She seemed to sense his sorrow.

He existed like this for three years before the predictable happened. He had awakened at 4:00 a.m. and slipped out of the house to walk the farm and check the water tanks and fences. A warm summer day was in the offing. He enjoyed the colorful sunrise over Mt. Hood.

"Gypsy, we're lucky to be here on this farm. It has been my salvation through all this," he said, showing the first small spark of interest in his surroundings. "Our flock of sheep over there don't realize how you protect them. I heard you barking the coyotes away last night. You take care of all of us, don't you, girl?"

Lovingly he scratched her head and then adjusted the float on a water tank. "I'll race you to the house," he said suddenly. A run made even more refreshing because of the clean mountain air. They ran full out. "We made it, girl," he said panting. "Thanks for letting me win."

It was 9:00 a.m. and the smell of bacon frying greeted him as he opened the kitchen door. "I see you're up and at 'em, Jill. I'm really hungry this morning. I hope the coffee's ready, it sure smells good."

"You are always out so early….I think that's what keeps you so fit. You never gain a pound and you love to eat."

The hard work on the farm agreed with Malcolm. Just yesterday he had chain sawed the last of the ten cords of wood they would use for winter. He had insisted on a wood furnace because he thought that kind of heat wrapped around you. He liked the smell of the sawdust that poured out from under the chain saw as it melted through a log. He had grown up enjoying the heat from a wood furnace and cook stove. Until he was about eight he watched his dad and then it was his job to keep the wood boxes filled. He loved the splitting and piling of wood in neat tight rows. He could look at it and think about a job well done.

His life was built on basics. He was grounded. He sat down at the breakfast table proud that Jill had been so fortunate to get dressed in that warmth that he had created when he tended the furnace before his morning walk. He drank coffee and tended her bacon, cooking on their kitchen wood stove.

"It was really brisk out there this morning but it's nice and cozy in here." Fall is not too far off is what he had intended to say next but all that came out was, "Fall is………."

Jill turned to see that Malcolm was in trouble. She ran over to him.

"My left arm tingles," were his last words. He went limp and silent. Drool ran from the corner of his mouth. He slumped forward over the table.

Jill placed a pillow from a nearby couch beneath his head. "Oh my God! Malcolm speak to me! Come on ……please…..speak to me!" She pleaded, "You're the strong one…don't do this to me."

Jill's stomach knotted. Helplessness consumed her. Her uncooperative fingers dialed 911. She bent over him and enclosed him in her arms to impart her love and transfuse life into him somehow.

A wailing siren came from afar and wound its way up the narrow road to the farm house. Two attendants lifted him onto a stretcher and placed an oxygen mask over his distorted face.

"His blood pressure is normal. He'll be okay," they reassured Jill. "You can follow in your car when you get ready. We'll take him to Providence Hospital."

She stood on the porch with Gypsy, crying, as the ambulance disappeared down the road. "It's okay, girl, he's okay…..I promise I'll bring him back to you."

Unfortunately, for Malcolm, strokes were considered untreatable at that time. Put the patient in bed and watch them. Watch one out of three die within 24 hours. The others could be gradually rehabilitated but would never recover completely.

A heart attack and a stroke are essentially the same disease but just a different organ is affected. Heart attacks always get more attention because the pump is more essential than the mind. We can survive with a severely damaged mind and/or paralysis.

This philosophy was well known by Dr. McKenna and he would be a very bad patient.

* * *

The chaplain approached his bed and tried to reassure him the next morning. "Doctor, you are very fortunate. You have an excellent physician in Doctor Saunders. He is doing everything available to modern science to help you."

"Yeah, he's giving me an aspirin," he wrote on his bedside clipboard. Fortunately it was his left side that was paralyzed and he could still use his right hand. He had always been totally right handed.

He requested that family members not visit. He did not want anyone to see him so helpless.

"Jill, tell everyone I'm okay and I'll see them later when I'm totally recovered," he wrote. He turned away from her. The pen moved again, "You don't need to waste your time here either. What can you do?"

Jill felt even more alone than she had these past few years. She was denied her obligation and her need to help her fallen warrior. She was now completely shut out of his life. "In his crusade to be invulnerable he is the most vulnerable of all," she thought.

Dr. Saunders stood at the foot of Malcolm's bed with chart in hand on the third hospital day. "I think you're depressed. I'll order some medication for that."

"No you won't. Of course I'm depressed. Wouldn't you be? Just get me out of this bed and I'll handle that depression," he scribbled angrily.

Dr. Saunders wrote orders for physiotherapy starting the next day. That order was usually given much later in a stroke as severe as this. Lab, x-ray and a complete cardiac work-up failed to show the cause. His blood pressure was normal. He was physically fit, not overweight and he had never smoked. His heart and arteries were remarkable for his age.

Dr. Saunders reported to Jill. "He's had a very severe stroke. We could not find the cause. Sometimes stress changes the body's chemistry, we believe. Physically he is very young for his age. His lungs are as healthy as any teenager, so we won't have to worry about pneumonia, the most common problem. He's so strong willed, I think he will do fine. He wants to be up already."

Malcolm's response to speech therapy was amazing. He was talking within three weeks. Tests on his mental dexterity were all normal. He had lost no cerebral cells because the blockage was in the brain stem and primarily affected his motor function. The loss was total, however, and he could not move his left arm or leg. Dr. Saunder's comment to Jill was ominous.

"He, in all probability, will never walk again, but his mind and memory should be normal in a short time."

"His mind has not been normal for some time now," she said carefully, still reeling from the doctor's just announced prognosis. "He has been so despondent. What can I do to help him?"

"That might explain why he had this stroke. I would recommend a psychiatrist. I'll talk to him. He has refused antidepressants."

"If I know him, he will refuse a psychiatrist too. He's as strong willed as a mule."

"That very fact may help him fight back now. You'll have to be patient. He has a long, long way to go. This is the ultimate insult to a man as physically active as he was."

Dr. McKenna remained in the hospital for five more weeks. He refused to let the nurses bathe him. Jill would push him in a special wheel chair into the spacious shower.

"I believe you're sitting up better each day," she said, as she sprayed the water over his waiting body. "Doesn't that warm water feel great?"

"No, it burns my left arm," he complained.

"It shouldn't burn you, it's barely warm."

"Don't tell me how I feel. It burns! You are always telling me how I feel."

"Sorry….but at least you're talking much better now," she tried to find something good to say. "Here, let me rub your back with this towel. I'll bet that feels good."

"Rub harder…right there…thanks. Jill, I have to get out of this place. That bed is so hard. Hour after hour I have to lie there in one spot. I can't turn you know." He looked directly into her eyes and asked, with such pain in his voice, "What use am I to you…or anybody now?"

"You have to ask? How can you not know how much you mean to me? You think a stroke makes the tiniest difference? You're still the same man I married, nothing has changed as far as I'm concerned." She smiled tenderly at him. "We'll just have to change our routine a little bit. Everything will be fine, you'll see." She pulled him close in her arms so he wouldn't see the tears streaming down her cheeks.

When she had recovered her composure she spoke quietly to the rest of his question. "Another thing, I'll need your medical knowledge to keep me well. We all do. The kids call me every day to see how you're doing. They know no little stroke can keep you down."

Bed had always been Malcolm's enemy. He used to jump up instantly in the morning to get away from it. He hated to waste time sleeping. "When you're in bed, you're dead," he would say. This hospital bed was getting revenge for all his years of bed hate. The mattress felt like the washboard his mother had used to torture his dirty clothes, before she got the Maytag. She hadn't seemed to mind that it had vibrated all over the back porch. One time, the ringer caught her hair when she was bending over it. Luckily she was able to reach the shut off switch or she would have been scalped. But his mother never complained. She lived such a simple life. He felt bad, looking back. He should have done much more to repay her for all those years she had devoted herself to him. Maybe she was watching over him now and he could at last ask her forgiveness. He had to try and now was as good a time as any. He began.

Please Forgive Me

Forgive me, mom
For not knowing
How small your world had become
After I had to take the car keys.

For not knowing your inner thoughts
At that moment.
I now think it was the first time that
I became your enemy.
I sensed it.
How could I not?
You said the only mean thing
You had ever said to me
In all those fifty years.
You said, "Your time will come."
You were right, mom, my time has come.
My world is becoming smaller and smaller.
My kids, like I then, don't see it.
They have their own busy lives to live.
I don't really fit.
My advice falls on deaf ears.
Forgive me, mom,
For not understanding why
You would always want to go back to that lonely house,
Early,
After I had picked you up for dinner with us.
I know now that lonely house was all
That was really yours.
You felt secure there.
You did not have the energy anymore to be social and patient
With the younger set. (Meaning us and your grandchildren).
You were the epitome of patience with me as I grew up,
And with your grandchildren after that.
You were like a Saint.
You always understood the foibles and fantasies of youth.

I should have understood that, and in return been patient with you.
I should have hired someone closer to your age to be your companion,
To drive you wherever you wanted to go.
Someone who could better understand your small world
Than I could.
I was too busy with the practice of medicine,
With the family,
And with knowing that life was really eternal,

To see that you knew more than I about that.
Money was not the problem, Mom,
I was just plain stupid about it.
I always loved you so much
But I couldn't say it.
Why?
Forgive me, Mom.

Even when you could no longer speak
You were able to say it
So clearly
That day I came to see you.

You had been in a coma
For days
You were dying slowly
But I know you weren't suffering any pain
Your reward
For being such a good person.

I leaned down
Over your pale, still body
And when my face
Was close to yours
You opened your eyes
For the last time and
Looked into my sad eyes
And you smiled.
The most beautiful smile
I have ever seen.
It said
I love you.
You did forgive me.

He must have been heard. He fell into a restful deep sleep. He had not slept that soundly since he entered the hospital.

"It's time for your therapy," Robin said in a cheerful voice. She and crew were there to lift him out of bed. He admired her, her hands were warm and caring. Her empathetic brown eyes reached deep inside him begging him to do the impossible. If anyone on earth could help him, he thought, it was Robin.

"You are much stronger today," she smiled. "You must have slept well." She encouraged his participation, "Here now, hold these bars. See, you're standing for the first time without my holding onto you."

She kneeled to push his left leg forward. "Your first step! Look at you! Who said you couldn't walk?" Her voice coaxed him along, "We'll show them."

He was embarrassed with such a feeble effort. "When I'm really walking I'll come back to see you, Robin. Yours is a noble calling. Do you know how important you really are?"

"I'll be here," Robin smiled warmly.

Back in that miserable bed, he tried to reassure himself that he would walk again one day. His kids and Jill needed him. Last night had made him realize that the answer was in deep thought. He must put himself into that peaceful trance state. No bed had ever existed there. He searched for pleasant thoughts long forgotten these past unhappy years. His mind drifted to Gabrielle, whom he had nicknamed Elle. She was in college now. She talked with him often about academia. He must help her find her place in life. She was still confused. What a joy she had always been. From the moment he delivered her and she rolled those big eyes at him, he was hooked. She reminded him of his mother. She had that same moral compass. She even liked the same food…..bacon, pork chops and oatmeal. She hated candy. He always joked that she was sweet enough without it anyway. She was fun to tease because she was always so literal.

She was six that Christmas morning. She had organized her gifts into a pile to be opened in some order that only she knew. She liked to prolong the process and talk about each item. She opened a delicately ribboned box that revealed a tiara. Jill thought she would like it because she was so taken with fairy princesses.

Malcolm quickly saw an opening. "Wow, that's really something, Elle……and I'll bet those are real diamonds too, look how they sparkle."

She went on with her plan without saying a word until almost five minutes had passed. She had given some thought to his comment and in all seriousness responded, "Dad, they could be rhinestones, you know." She was the princess that Jill helped create. She and her mother were very much alike. Both were tall, beautiful, intelligent and proud. Elle was a lot like him too. She was stubborn and deep.

Elle was never the farm hand he had hoped for. She was in no sense a tomboy. She hated the smell of manure and never stepped a foot into the chicken house. She was too afraid of the aggressive rooster who resided there. Even Jill could not muster up enough courage to face up to him. Elle did enjoy the clean hay up in the loft, however. She liked its sweet fresh smell and the complete freedom of being carefree and alone.

One summer day, when she was twelve, she felt courageous enough to venture some distance from the house and take her cat for a walk. This was the Siamese/Ragdoll that she had always dressed up in her old doll's clothing. It slept in pajamas on her bed. These two were alike and definitely urbanites.

They walked downhill where a wooded area to the south provided enough darkness to be somewhat foreboding. They stayed inside the fence that protected them but when they came to the farthest corner the cat tired and cried to be picked up. Elle carried her through the tall grass toward the house. In the middle of the field, they heard a loud ominous snort. Elle and her companion were petrified with fear. Grass parted in all directions as she began to run, faster and faster up the hill. The cat was hugged tightly against her side by its neck, its tail and leash flying straight out behind her with the speed of her flight. She was gasping for breath when she finally set her down.

Dad confronted her at the top of the hill. "Why the hurry, kid? You ran up that hill in twenty seconds flat."

She was breathing so hard, she could hardly get the words out. "I heard a wild boar! It was attacking us!" She was shaking.

"There are no wild boars here," he reassured her. "It must have been a buck deer. They will snort if you surprise them and get too close. Remember how I always used to call those loud smelly mistakes people sometimes make, *bucksnorts*? Well, that's the story behind that."

* * *

He found solace and escape from sleepless nights on the ever harder, more confining prison of his hospital bed. By recalling his children's fun times he was able, for a little while, to transport himself back to happier days.

After Elle, his youngest, he thought about James, his oldest, who had been born at the medical school. He thought first about the medical emergency, an alarming experience when a rubber tire from a toy car got lost up his nose. Later on, at the farm, wheels would be much bigger when James developed a passion for motorcycles. This was the doctor's nightmare because he had treated so many broken heads from crashes. He compromised with his son by extracting a promise that he would never ride on the asphalt and compete with traffic. They constructed a dirt bike trail on the farm.

James fished a little but enjoyed bow hunting more. He shot his first buck in the Wallowas hunting with his dad, long before Jill had enjoyed "Little Switzerland." James was also a dependable farm hand and loved driving the tractor. They hayed together every summer. All the kids loved to ride on the hay wagon when it was loaded and on the trip to the barn. They always felt high and mighty way up on top, and they were, literally mighty high. There was a large caliber rope tied to the barn rafters. The kids played Tarzan in the hay. Malcolm, on one trip down from the field, grabbed that rope and yelled at the top of his voice as he swung from the hay trailer. The kids were all surprised and feared that he had gone berserk. But it made him feel free and very young again, like they were.

He was still swinging through the air when breakfast awakened him. He could not chew so the food was liquid and tiresome. He had a little trouble swallowing too, so it was a slow unpleasant process. He was losing weight and he had little to spare. The entire daytime routine was a bummer and he longed for lights out when he could think his own thoughts and dream without interruption.

His other sons, Sean and Stewart, were a pair of opposites. Sean was born during his Seattle internship and remained "big city", always. He hated the farm and was alienated from his brothers, Stewart and James. They paired off to work hard and ride their motor cycles. He was a stylish dresser when he wasn't lying on the deck sunbathing. Malcolm never did understand Sean and often thought about what his father had said when he saw Sean in the hospital nursery.

"That boy skins a bad eye, you'll have trouble with him."

Malcolm was mystified by his father's frequent proclamations but that one topped them all. What could anyone see in a baby's eyes? Nonetheless, he and Sean were never close. The most one on one time he ever had with him was that trip to Sun Valley soon after his marriage to Jill. He was surprised that Sean wanted to go but Sean and Jean were much closer. The three of them had enjoyed the snow that Christmas. Sean was tall and slender and enjoyed track and skiing. He was very bright and very much the practical joker. Malcolm understood that part of him best, but came away from the trip still not connected. His sense of humor had an arrogance about it that left Malcolm unimpressed.

Stewart must have sensed it too and stayed close to James even though they were farther apart in age and different in many ways. James was Grandpa McKenna's favorite, perhaps because they were so much alike. Both were salt of the earth, steady as you go, dependable. They were fun to be around. Stewart was less talkative and substituted a ready knowing smile for grandpa's pleasant verbosity. He used his brilliant insight to be quick on the trigger. He couldn't wait to grow up and enjoy his older brother's trail blazing spirit.

Malcolm remembered suturing Stewart's chin when he had fallen against the fireplace as a toddler. He could still see the frightened look on James' face when he reported that Stewart was lying on the steep wooded trail where he had fallen from his bike. That fear was deep concern about his brothers broken leg and also because his doctor dad had predicted such a disaster. The doctor examined the leg and splinted it and then the dad carried Stewart up out of the ravine.

His office x-ray pronounced the leg normal. The dad's two sons were more in awe of the man they lived with. They felt his compassion and his power.

"It's 7:30, you were sleeping so soundly I hated to wake you." Malcolm opened his eyes knowing he must walk again. His family would always need him. Their problems were more complex now, but he was more understanding.

Robin was amazed at how hard Malcolm was trying. The mental vibrations were almost palpable. Could such strong signals coming down somehow bypass the short circuit? She knew they would.

"Malcolm, I know you will walk again. It's just a matter of time. Here let me help," she offered. She was sure she felt an imperceptible movement. The left foot was sliding ever so slowly forward.

"Hold that thought……..make it grow…" She lifted the foot again and again.

That afternoon Malcolm was confronted with another problem. Dr. Fields, a urologist, introduced himself. "I'm Dr. Fields. Dr. Saunders wanted me to see you. Your blood work showed an elevated PSA."

"What's a PSA?"

"It's a new blood test for prostate cancer. It should be below 2. Yours is 14.4."

"I have prostate cancer?"

"We'll have to check it out. I've never seen one that high."

Dr. Fields did a rectal exam. "It is enlarged but it feels soft. I'll set you up for an ultrasound examination tomorrow."

When Jill came in soon after, he confessed. "Guess what? I don't need to have any more physiotherapy. I have the big C."

"You mean cancer? Are you kidding me?"

"No, Dr. Fields was in today. He will confirm it with an ultrasound and biopsy tomorrow."

"I can't believe this. You were fine before the stroke."

"I can't believe it either. Maybe it's a false alarm."

This turn of events hit Malcolm hard. He went numb and slept very little that night. The test the next day was painful. About six or seven biopsies were taken and each one was some kind of spring-loaded explosion deep inside. He was in a cold sweat from worry and from pain. Jill worried along with him. She had had a fitful night of anguish, too.

"It's been three days. When will we get the pathology report?"

"Maybe today……….I hope."

It was about an hour later and Jill was still there when Dr. Fields showed up. "I've got some good news. The biopsy report is negative."

"How do you account for such a false alarm then? I haven't slept and I stopped my PT. This is crazy."

"I understand why you're so upset Dr. McKenna. This is a new test and I guess we don't completely understand it. This was definitely a false positive."

"Thanks for your concern. I know you were just doing your job."

Dr. Fields left the room. Jill was irate. "What kind of nonsense was all this? You didn't need such a scare. This was the worst possible timing."

"You and I both know that doctors are frequently their own worst enemies. They love exact science. They worship blood tests and common sense goes out the window. This PSA, like the PBI thyroid fiasco, is going to do a lot of harm……..I hope it does some good in the process. If I were still practicing, I would have put it on the back burner for sure. The only time a blood test should be ordered is to substantiate a diagnosis you have made by the history and physical exam. Blood tests and x-rays are expensive and usually unnecessary. I would never have ordered this test."

Malcolm was so worn out that he fell asleep long before lights out. It was a fitful sleep, but he had pleasant dreams once again.

Jean was his second child and his first daughter. He protected her and spoiled her. She was always a joy. She loved her father as much as he loved her. She tried hard to please him. She worked part-time in his office from age twelve until she graduated from college. She and Elle were the best receptionists he ever had. They were very efficient and at the same time, warm and people-oriented. A rare combination.

Jean loved horses and farm life but her younger sister, Bree, was perhaps the greatest animal lover of them all. She spent much of her time with a baby chicken or other newborn in her lap. She grew up to become a vegetarian because she couldn't bear the thought of any animal being killed.

When Bree wasn't outside she loved to bake cookies and delighted in watching her father eat them. He always told her they were the best he had ever tasted. She was very studious and he helped her with home work. It was math that irritated her most. Jean told him later that Bree was the smartest of the clan. When she grew up, Bree lived on a few acres with more than a few animals. He knew he was needed there for sure.

Jean traveled and worked on a cruise ship for about ten years and then moved back to the Glen Oak farm in Sandy that he had vacated. She lives there still with all her beloved animals. He must walk again to visit and help her manage it. Thinking back over those early years he remembered how devastated she had been when the milkman ran over her little poodle, Migi. He foolishly tried to fix the problem by bringing home a new puppy. It was the basset hound he had always wanted and not the proper dog for a delicate little girl. She sensed that his heart was in the right place and overlooked the faux pas. She tried hard to love Sam, a big, lumbering, slobbering oaf of a dog. He would follow her school bus and embarrass her.

She was riding home with her father one day from school and during their conversation, innocently threw in the "f" word that she had heard some boys using.

"Jean," Malcolm said matter of factly, but gently, "Nice girls, like you, never use that word. It's not acceptable." She knew her daddy was always right so she was very careful from that day forward to never use that word or any other slang again. She grew up to be a polite and considerate, lovable woman, and he was always proud of her.

She accompanied him on a trip to the University of Mexico medical school in Mexico City when she was sixteen. Some fellow travelers, on a tour bus there, complimented him on his beautiful wife. He thought about it for a few minutes before he replied, "She is a beauty, but my wife is much younger.......this is my sister."

* * *

"Time to have breakfast," Robin gently prodded. "You're going home today! We have to get you dressed."

As much as he had waited for this day he was not happy to have that wonderful trip to Mexico interrupted.

"My, you do sleep well. Tell me your secret."

"It's my innocence I guess. I only think kind thoughts about people. Even you," he joked.

He was ready and waiting in the wheelchair when Jill arrived. He said his goodbyes down the hall at physiotherapy. Robin hugged him and made him promise to come back for a visit.

"I will walk in here pushing this wheelchair before you know it," he laughed.

Chapter XXXI

The Long Road Back

Riding in the car, home from the hospital, was a thrill. He enjoyed seeing the houses and all the people going about their normal routines. He thought all that had stopped because he had stopped.

Dale, the farm hand, helped lift Malcolm out of the car into the wheelchair. Gypsy ran from the porch to greet him. She put her head in his lap, as usual, and wailed that soulful moan. He scratched her neck with his useful right hand. He saw himself out of that chair, running with her as before.

"She hasn't left the porch all the time you were gone. She did come over to the barn a few times when she heard me, but as soon as she didn't see you she walked directly back to her bed there," Dale informed him.

He sat there with Gypsy for almost two hours looking around outside at the garden and fence lines that he had walked each day. He now became painfully aware of his paralysis. To walk out there on the uneven ground was more of a challenge than he could bear. He knew he would never cross those fences again. He was stuck without those wheels.

He cried and held onto Gypsy for moral support. "Somehow we'll get out there together, you and I."

Jill came out to push him into the house. "I hope you're not addicted to that hospital food. I've cooked your favorite meal, roast beef with mashed potatoes and gravy."

"Sure does smell good, Jill. Looks good in here too. Let's have a fire in the fireplace tonight. God, it's good to be home."

Jill had to cut his meat but he ate like he was making up for lost time. He was down twenty-five pounds since the stroke.

She was relieved to see he had his old appetite back. "I'll let you order the menu for a while. Just tell me what you're hungry for and I'll fix it."

"That's why I married you, for your cooking, and I'll let you have your way just this once."

Jill went to sleep that night happy to see his dramatic change in attitude. His sense of humor was back at last. She had always appreciated his quickness to see the funny side of most anything when you least expected it.

Malcolm was forced to sleep on a portable bed downstairs because he couldn't manage the long steep stairway up to their bedroom. He had always shared a bed with Jill. He needed her warm body close to him, especially now. Jill had never known how much Malcolm's invincibility depended on her. This was his fault, and now he saw that flaw in his character. He would endure his punishment because he had no choice; it was too late to do otherwise.

Jill's "looks don't last, but cookin' do" attitude was at least half right. In his mind the only way out was to become physically and mentally strong again. It was a cruel trick that fate had played on him. He was not impotent….that fact would do battle with the rest of him and demand constant attention. He didn't know how to deal from weakness. This was exactly the attitude he needed to rehabilitate himself.

The deck on the west side of the house was wheel chair accessible. He would wheel himself out there to enjoy the sunrises and view across the farm. Gypsy was always there when she heard the door open. His goal was to find a way to walk the length of that long narrow outside world. Its thirty-foot length was smooth, inviting and remotely possible.

Jill would help him out of the chair and hold him while he got his balance which was a tremendous effort for him. A cold sweat was his constant companion at these times. His powerful mind had to ignore his body constantly telling him "I can't." The left foot slid forward a few inches at a time.

After three weeks he took a feeble step. Jill applauded like a mother would, watching her baby do the same. He hated that simile but he knew walking was one step at a time and he would suffer any indignity to accomplish that end.

It helped him to think back over recent progress. When they lifted him out of bed for the first two or three weeks at the hospital he could not hold himself in a sitting position in a chair. Pillows were used around him to keep him upright. He recalled the first time he was pulled to a standing position from the wheelchair. The room was spinning around him and he became nauseated.

Now that he could stand for a short time he would concentrate on his foot. It looked normal. It had to move. He was sure a few months from now he would look back at this feeble effort and use those thoughts to prod himself to even greater heights. He had no choice. This was all he had going for him.

Impatience was his enemy, he must control it. He tried and when no one was looking, he cried. He was embarrassed for Jill to see him struggling so hard. He knew that it was his strength and resilience that had captured her heart. Now that he had no strength, he must be resilient. He was, and that would save him.

He could see that the foot needed some kind of constant stimulation. Those intermittent deck walking fiascos were never going to work. He sat in their antique rocking chair one day and suddenly realized that he could make every part of him, including that left foot, move. His right leg powered the entire sequence. He smiled and rocked faster and faster. He could feel his left foot pushing against the floor, over and over again.

"That's it......I can rock that stupid foot right out of its dumb disconnect. I'll show it who's boss." He rocked by the hour, thinking about the old sea captain who had owned the chair originally over a hundred years ago. Longing for a ship and longing to walk again, had a lot in common.

It felt good to move again.

"I'm surprised you don't rock yourself to sleep," Jill observed.

"I'm not rocking myself asleep, I'm rocking myself awake," he joked.

Jill was amazed that the deck walks began to be for real. He began to move at last. He could take five or six steps before total exhaustion stopped him. Those few steps were questionably psychokinetic. No matter, they were steps and within a few weeks he could walk to the far edge of the deck.

"You are doing already what the doctor said you would never do. I'm so impressed," Jill said encouragingly.

"That's music to my ears, Jill, but we're just getting started."

Jill thought back to the birth of Gabrielle and how confident and in control he had been. He was beginning to sound like that man again. She hugged him with joy in her heart.

She drove him to the therapy pool in NW Portland twice a week. He was thrilled to see how much better his leg moved in the warm water. He would go from one side of the pool to the other, hopping and splashing. He stood out from the other stroke victims who had been coming there much longer, some for over a year. The therapist was in total disbelief that his stroke had been so recent.

His goal was to be able to get up onto his John Deere. He knew he could grade the road and do some other worthwhile chores from up on that tractor seat. It was power steering so he could handle it with one hand. Jill was petrified at the thought of him up so high on such a powerful vehicle. She reassured herself that he would not be able to fulfill that strong desire anytime soon so she put the whole nightmare out of her mind.

His other stated goal was to navigate the stairway to the bedroom. To lift his left leg up one step at a time was all he had to do he thought. He hung onto the railing with his good right hand and dared his left foot to come with him. "If you don't cooperate, I'll go up without you," he warned.

He tried over and over again, day after day, then after a few weeks… ."Jill, come quick and see where I am," he said proudly.

"You're halfway up those steps! How in the world did you do that?" She ran to stand on the step just below him, "Let me stand here, in front of you, and help you back down……you'll break in a million pieces if you fall," she said, fearing for him.

"Tonight I'll make it all the way to the top and sleep in my bed."

He did just that and his reward was worth the monumental effort. A few weeks later he coaxed Dale to help him up onto the tractor seat. Now he had real wheels. He drove it around until dark. He shouted to the heavens at the top of his voice, "I'm a free man now. I have power."

Dale delivered him safely back to the house where Jill was waiting anxiously for his return. "You will have an accident if you go too fast," Jill said, worry evident in her voice. "And it could tip over if you're not careful. Are you sure this is a good idea?" She liked it better when she could keep track of him in the house.

"Jill, you always were a worry wart." He hoped by stressing the obvious he could ease her apprehension, "I've driven a tractor for forty plus years. I'll be careful, okay?"

When the hospital found out about his unheard of progress, they sent out a photographer and an article appeared in their monthly magazine chronicling his phenomenal comeback.

"Jill, this gives me an idea. I can help all those depressed new stroke victims. Let's buy a wooden rocking chair like mine and put a plaque on it.

They can use it in the rehab department. He designed the plaque to read, "Shine don't whine……Rock yourself back." Directly beneath the message was a simple design of the sun with radiating lines to depict the brightness of their futures. Hundreds of stroke victims overcame their depressions in that chair. Helping others again was helping him too.

* * *

In the early 1900s their farm had been a dairy. The barn built at that time was oversized and the floor was constructed with thick cedar planks. It had been dismantled in the fifties and those planks stockpiled. Malcolm had used them to build a goat shed and a pig pen. He had always been frugal in saving usable lumber. These expensive rare cedar planks would have another unexpected calling at this point in his life.

He sat on his tractor and used the hydraulic bucket to move them to a level area behind the farm house. Dale sawed them to fit three raised beds, with easily accessed walkways between. Malcolm used the bucket to fill them with rich, high humus soil from the wooded area near the south pasture. Scoops of barnyard manure were layered at the bottom on heavy duty plastic for weed control. He was an expert at using the levers that controlled the hydraulic bucket; he had learned to master all that with his right hand. Now he was set up to garden despite his disability.

He and Gypsy spent many summertime hours there; planting, watering and watching vegetables grow. He knew that his organic produce would help him recover and the sense of accomplishment would be as important as the nutrition.

He was in the garden one morning when a dove flew down and landed on his shoulder. He never understood how it knew where he was because the dove pen was a block away, on the far side of the house. On occasion that dove would escape the enclosure when the door was opened. It would sit in a tree, watching him, and he could coax it back inside with food. He was addicted to their plaintive cooing call. He had first heard that sound along the river where he grew up. It had always been a part of his love for the outdoors. The call of the wild dove. It soared above all the other sounds and spoke to his heart.

Within a year after the stroke, he was hobbling around the farm with only a cane to help him. He and Gypsy were taking their walks once again.

"We can't hop fences anymore but its more fun opening gates anyway."

He carried on a constant conversation with her. Gypsy sensed how fragile his balance was and was careful not to get too close. She would wait until he was seated and stable to nuzzle him. She had become a self-trained guard dog.

Looking out over the valley below, he was dreaming about better days. "I won't be able to hunt again," he reminisced aloud. "I did a Hollywood style hunt over in southeastern Oregon up on Hart Mountain, Gypsy, did I ever tell you about that?" He reached to pet her, "You should have been there with me. My friend, Bill Barnes came up from L.A. with a professional photographer. We met there to make a documentary called, "Of Men and Muskets", and the camera man, Dave, gave me a hat to wear. He said it had belonged to John Wayne. It was one that he had worn in several movies and Dave thought it would look good on me. Think of that…..me in John Wayne's hat." He stroked Gypsy's head absentmindedly as he continued. "He said it would look great with the buckskins I was wearing…..It really was some kind of outfit; leather pants and soft Indian-style fringed boots………" He rambled on, letting his thoughts carry him back and he was once again on location. "I'll never forget how Dave posed me for that still shot."

"'Up there' Dave said, motioning to me, 'See that opening between the bush and the craggy tree? Stand there.' Then he positioned my legs just so, told me where to look and how to hold my old muzzle loader. When it all came together it was pretty spectacular if I do say so myself. We still have that picture somewhere and Jill has always loved it. She thinks it's one of the best pictures of me ever taken, John Wayne's hat and all. Gypsy, I don't know if you're aware of it, but Jill is becoming quite an artist. She's studying portrait painting and when she gets good enough she wants to paint that picture of me. That would be something, wouldn't it girl?" Gypsy hung on his every word as if she really understood.

Fall was approaching and the blackberries were ripening. They grew to make a fifteen foot wall along the south boundary of the farm where it met a wooded glen. Malcolm had always prized those berries, especially the big juicy ones that grew near the top. He had in the past, picked pails full on his early morning walks. Jill enjoyed them on her corn flakes. He had always felt so proud contributing to those special breakfasts.

When he came in, bearing the first berries of the season, Jill would always act surprised. She never failed to comment on how much she loved them and how clever he was to be able to find the perfect ones, so big and juicy.

Now he stood there, looking up at the prize. He would never be able to get them again.

He spotted Dale by the barn and called out, "Dale, could you bring that tall stepladder up here?"

"I don't think you should use that now……do you want me to pick for you?" he asked hopefully.

"No, just lean the ladder into the bushes over there." He managed to climb a few steps with Dale looking on. "See……I'm okay. You can get back to whatever you were doing and thanks." Dale left him reluctantly. He knew that when Malcolm had a mindset he had to go along with it.

Malcolm reached the prize berries and had the bucket about half full when he lost his balance and fell backwards onto the hard ground. He blacked out for a few minutes and awakened with Gypsy licking his face. "Did we spill the berries, girl? Maybe you'd better go get Dale to help me up."

Gypsy returned shortly with Dale in tow. "You're lucky this time, Doc. No broken bones I hope."

"Dale, you're sworn to secrecy. Jill must never know about this…… word of honor?"

He presented Jill the handful of berries that had somehow remained intact. "It's the beginning of the season," he said apologetically, "there will be more next time."

"Oh, but they are beautiful. How on earth did you pick them? I know the first ripe ones are at the very top."

"I'll never tell you that secret. I have to be able to do at least one thing that you can't."

* * *

A few months later, when winter had iced everything over, he had another bad experience. Jill had gone to the store never dreaming he would venture out on a day like that. She always underestimated him. He put on his heavy sheepskin coat and was headed around the house to the furnace room. He wanted to fill the fireplace pass-through. He loved to watch the fire and kept it alive all winter.

A few steps on the ice convinced him he had made a mistake. He tried to turn back, but his feet flew out from under him and he found himself lying flat on his back. The cold east wind was blowing mercilessly over him. Gypsy sat on his chest licking his face.

"I know you mean well, girl, but I'll never be able to get up with you on top of me." He pushed her off and slid himself downhill to the split rail fence that surrounded the back yard. He struggled to pull himself up with his strong right arm. His cheeks and hands were red and smarting from the relentless wind. He hugged the fence back to the porch.

"Gypsy, we made it just in time. Jill will be back any moment now," he remarked, pleased to have gotten away, unscathed and undetected, with this latest escapade.

Jill found him seated by the fire rubbing his cold hands. "You're red as a beet……What happened?"

"Oh, I needed some fresh air and stayed out on the porch with Gypsy too long. She really didn't want me to leave her," he smiled innocently.

Chapter XXXII

Healing the Soul

The upstairs bedroom in the farm house was an architectural wonder. Hops, an essential ingredient for fine beer, thrived in the Willamette Valley. Malcolm grew up admiring the twenty-five foot vines that climbed strings held high by endless rows of wooden posts supporting overhead wires. A twenty-acre hop field rising dramatically in the distance would tower above fields of grass or even corn. To him, it had a kind of poetic symmetry. Man made the frame and nature painted the living picture.

He recalled one drive through the countryside when he had spotted a strange building on an abandoned hop farm. The building was windmill shaped and rose high above the house. It was sided with shingles, had a small entry door at ground level and multi-paned windows near the top. He could not imagine the purpose of what appeared to be a down scaled version of the Washington Monument in DC. He later learned that it had been a hop dryer.

Bringing those memories together with his other love for a cupola he had seen somewhere in his travels, he designed the bedroom. It was like a second building placed high atop the rambling first floor. The sides were sloping and capped with a quasi cupola four-sided roof. From inside you looked up sixteen feet into the peak. Six foot triangular stained glass windows, depicting the four seasons, capped the large picture windows directly beneath. From the bed one could look out in all directions at the breathtaking view. He felt like an eagle in it's' nest.

Jill set up her easel in one corner of that rustic grandeur. The ambiance was perfect for a budding artist. Malcolm knew that true artistic ability was inherited. He had none. This perspective enabled him to see Jill's potential long before she could. Her progress was natural and effortless.

He promoted her talent passionately. This was something he could do while sitting to rest his tired leg. He had too much time to spare in that regard. Jill was unaware of his plan to see that she would become world renowned.

Early into the fourth year of her endeavor, she surprised him by announcing, "I'm ready to paint the hunter on Hart Mountain." The photograph was the standard 2x3 inches and her canvas 24x30. This was going to be a real statement and Malcolm was pleased. Before long the rifle-bearing frontiersman gradually began to take form. He could see the progress every morning when he awoke. It was as though he vicariously was the painter and his admiration for Jill grew with the painting. He was formulating intricate plans to cast sunlight on Jill's shadowed talent.

Malcolm belonged to a group called *Young Americas*, whose mission was to expose young people to common sense and help temper youthful idealism. Service in the Second World War had helped him shake that disease, idealism, of youth in short order. He wanted those that followed him to have a less painful experience.

Young Americas had recently been influential in purchasing President Ronald Reagan's ranch near Santa Barbara. The goal was to preserve, intact, that Western White House. The fact that President Reagan had a ranch outlet, where he could charge his batteries, so to speak, appealed to Malcolm. He had done the same through all his hectic years of medical practice.

Jill and Malcolm had been the privileged recipients of a private tour of Rancho del Cielo a few years earlier. "That was one of the most memorable days of my life," he repeated many times later. He had seen firsthand the fences and trails built by the famous president. Riding boots and bathrobe hung in the closet of the small adobe bungalow the Reagans affectionately knew as their home away from The White House. It was as though the President still lived there and would arise and put them on in the morning and go about the business of the day. His presence was heavy and permeated the air. It was hard to believe he would never again return. President Reagan was incapacitated by the ravages of Altzheimer's Disease. He was unaware that he had been President or ever owned that ranch in the sky. Malcolm was thankful his own mind had been spared.

Jill, at last, finished the Hart Mountain painting. It seemed a miracle to Malcolm how that little photograph had been transferred so life-like onto canvas. He was proud to be the subject and to be the husband of the artist. They hung it in the place of honor over the fireplace.

"You've arrived, Jill……..that is an absolute masterpiece!" Everyone who saw it agreed. He was now more eager than he had ever been, to follow up on his grand plan to promote Jill.

Many years earlier, in San Francisco, he had read a very thin book one afternoon. He was staying at the house of a friend and business associate. That fateful afternoon his friend was downtown at his office and Malcolm had a few hours to kill until dinner that night. He went into the library looking for something to read. There it was at eye level, lying on a book shelf. It was so thin he almost missed it. Someone was obviously reading it and had laid it there, out of place.

A prediction from the *Celestine Prophecy* had already come true. He had picked up the book almost handed to him by chance, in a library in San Francisco, where he was visiting by chance. He read the confusing book before dinner. It was the kind of quick read that you think about later more than you do at the moment. He carried away the idea that everyone you meet and every situation in which you find yourself can be important. You have to be aware that opportunity often knocks only once and you may have to listen carefully to hear the faint sound of it.

The plan he had in mind not only entailed being aware of an opportunity but setting up the situation for the opportunity to occur. This may sound complicated, and it is, but Malcolm was very good at making things happen. Experience had taught him that no one is looking out for you, except you. He didn't have to wait long. It arrived in the mail a few short days after they had placed the painting Jill named *Of Men and Muskets* over the fireplace.

"Look at this, Jill, we've been invited to London with a group from *Young Americas*. They want to explore how Winston Churchill's country estate, Chartwell, is being presented to the public and preserved for posterity."

"You're reading that with such enthusiasm…...are you considering that we will go?" Jill knew how impossible international travel would be for Malcolm. They had taken very few short, local trips since his stroke.

"Churchill has always been one of my heroes and I'm not about to miss such an opportunity."

"Let's think about it. What is the RSVP date?"

"It's next month. The trip is planned for this fall." Malcolm knew they had to go, but now was not the time to push. "You're right, we'll sleep on it."

About a week later, he was talking to Elle on the phone. "We're going to London in September. Do you want to go along?" He invited her, knowing how much she loved a new adventure. He would need her travel expertise and even her physical support, plus she was just plain fun to be around. Jill and Elle were equally amazed, but felt it would be cruel to talk him out of it.

The flight from Portland to LA to New York to London's Heathrow would be difficult for anyone; for Malcolm it was a nightmare. When they checked into their room at the Savoy, he collapsed on the bed. "Give me a few minutes before we go out on the town." The laughter that filled the room was hysterical. They were all exhausted.

The next morning at breakfast they agreed that the world famous Savoy was stodgy and too British. "This is a perfect headquarters for the stuffy meetings, Dad." Elle spread the many maps she had picked up on their way through the hotel lobby across the bed. "I have some great tours planned for our free time. We'll see London and the British Museum today." Elle was the enthusiastic guide Malcolm had known she would be.

The main event was scheduled for mid week. Chartwell was about three hours outside of London. The estate loomed majestically above the rolling green pastures. It was not a house but a veritable mansion built in the 14th century. It could not be compared to President Reagan's remodeled bungalow at Rancho del Cielo. Knights of the roundtable rather than cowboys of the old west. Malcolm sat in the library where Churchill had pondered those eloquent speeches. His mind whirred back in time. He felt the presence of his hero.

Churchill's granddaughter, Celia Sandys, was there to greet them. She was a charming hostess and she gave him an autographed copy of the new book she had just completed, *Churchill Wanted Dead or Alive.*

On the ride back to London, he thought about the clock. Turn it back and he could have visited Churchill at Chartwell and traveled this road to London with him. The experience of these past few hours was a monumental privilege. With effort and imagination, the clock can be turned back.

The trip was climaxed by a final meeting in a spacious conference room at the Savoy. Everyone had a chance to talk about the significance of the past few days and how they felt about Young Americas.

Malcolm's comment was sincere. "I want to thank you for inviting us to share this journey. It has been most rewarding and we will take away many good memories of new friends and shared experiences. I deem it a real privilege to be a part of this fine organization. Ours is a noble cause.

I will never forget these past few days and I know they will help us see a direction for Rancho Del Cielo. Again, and I speak for myself and my family here with me, thank you one and all."

An aura of the Celestine Prophecies hung heavy over the small anteroom near the main conference hall where Elle, Jill and Malcolm waited expectantly, seated in soft easy chairs. Malcolm had requested a private meeting with Ron Robinson, president of *Young Americas*. The headquarters of this organization was near Washington DC, so Malcolm seldom had such an opportunity to confer in person with the top echelon. Ron came in and sat down. After the usual small talk, Malcolm turned the conversation to the subject he had been waiting to introduce.

"Ron, Elle lives in L.A. near Santa Barbara," he began. "I was hoping she could be helpful in some way with the Reagan Ranch Museum."

"I'm sure she would be a valuable resource for us," Ron responded. "I'll keep it in mind." More small talk ensued to include Jill's portrait painting.

Malcolm's enthusiasm was palpable. Here was a subject that was near and dear to his heart. "She just finished a masterpiece called *Of Men and Muskets*," he said proudly. "The name comes from a documentary I made years ago," he added as a point of interest. "She painted me from a snapshot she admired that was taken during that shoot."

Ron listened attentively to Malcolm extolling his wife's accomplishments. When he seemed to have reached his conclusion, Ron turned to face Jill. "Jill, would you consider a portrait of President Reagan? We could use one painted from a snapshot we have of him at the ranch for the museum in Santa Barbara."

"It would be an honor; she would love to do it." Malcolm spoke quickly before Jill had a chance to respond. Later, in the privacy of their room, she had some harsh words for her benefactor. "Do you realize what you've done?" She was panicking. "I'm an amateur.......not a professional. Paint the President of the United States? Oh my God!"

"You are not an amateur. Your paintings don't lie. You are going to be famous," he stated flatly. "I have no doubts."

Three weeks later a registered manila envelope arrived from Ron Robinson's DC office. He formally commissioned her to do the portrait. Two 8 x 10 photographs soon followed from the ranch museum. She was asked to select one. She chose a pose of him taken in front of the rail fence he had built. A cowboy hat and detailed plaid shirt insured that it would be much more difficult to paint, but also more appropriate for the museum.

She chose a 3 x 4 foot canvas. This would be the largest portrait she had ever attempted. To properly proportion the painting she needed to extend his body downward, almost to his knees. The photograph had cut him off just above the belt line. She requested photographs of some of his buckles and they sent her a dozen of his favorites. She selected a simple silver one that spelled out his name with chips of turquoise.

She labored over the canvas for almost a full year. Malcolm thought it was finished after about seven months. He should have known that to an artist a painting is never really finished to their satisfaction. They always see minor changes that have to be made.

To his surprise, one Sunday morning, she carried it down stairs and propped it up on the kitchen counter top, announcing, "It's finished!" Her eyes reflected triumph and anticipation. What would people think of it?

A surge of emotion welled up in Malcolm's throat and for a moment he was unable to speak. His stomach was knotted with pride and when he spoke his voice was unsteady. "It looks like he could step right off that canvas and shake my hand" he observed. "His facial expression seems to be one of complete satisfaction. Follow his gaze….I think he was looking out toward the field where his horses were grazing……..He really loved that ranch and it shows in his face, don't you think?"

"I agree with what you're saying. I get exactly the same feeling. I think I'm going to name it *Peace of Mind*. That pretty much says it all, wouldn't you say?"

"Jill, I have goose bumps right now." He rubbed his arm just thinking about it. "Do you realize that's the only painting like it in the world? We have to protect it until we can deliver it to Santa Barbara."

The final framed version was a massive 4 x 5 feet. Jill and Malcolm both felt strongly that the frame needed to be something really unusual and very special to honor this man and his celebrated ranch. It had been, after all, the western Whitehouse, visited by Gorbachev, Margaret Thatcher and even the Queen of England. Jill designed a unique frame made of clear Oregon Ponderosa pine with an imbedded hemp rope. A specialty wood working shop and framer were utilized to cut it. The frame by itself was a work of art.

"We'll drive down to L.A. for a visit with Elle. We can drop the painting off in Santa Barbara on the way. I can't trust any shipper with this treasure," Malcolm announced with pride.

"That will be a fun trip," Jill agreed to the plan.

The curator, Marilyn, was genuinely thrilled when the painting was unwrapped. She showed them some other portraits of the President stored in a back room. It was obvious that *Peace of Mind* was in a class by itself. Their presence was requested at the unveiling that would take place two weeks later at the yearly VIP meeting of *Young Americas*.

Jill's adulation began when they entered the door that night. The girl that was registering the guests recognized her name. "Oh my gosh….. you're the artist! Your painting has created quite a stir around here. It's absolutely magnificent!"

When *Peace of Mind* was unveiled by Jill, the 300 in attendance simultaneously exhaled a plauditory…."oh!!!!!" President Ron Robinson moved closer to get a better look. "My God," he said softly, "it's priceless!" He kissed her on the cheek, which was totally unexpected from the stoic Ron. He busied himself then, pulling the folding chairs away from the wall where the painting hung. He too, was feeling that need to protect it. Malcolm stood back and watched the procession of people congratulating Jill. His was a satisfied, knowing smile.

Peter Robinson had written a new book, *How Ronald Reagan Changed My Life*. He was the key speaker that evening. He had been one of President Reagan's speech writers and had a part in the writing of the memorable Berlin Wall speech. When he handed Jill a signed copy of his book, he shook her hand.

"It is a pleasure to shake the hand that painted such a likeness of President Reagan. I have seen all the paintings of him up close. Yours is by far the best. You've really captured the essence of the man." Jill still hadn't recovered by the time they started their drive back home early the next morning.

"Didn't I tell you so?" Malcolm gloated.

"Yes, you did. Now I believe you, but I'll need a little more adoration here……I'm having withdrawal," she laughed.

That portrait of President Reagan would change their lives. Jill was commissioned by many people of note. She became well-known and very busy. Malcolm remained her greatest fan and promoter.

Now that Jill was famous in her own right, he needed to reinvent himself. He hoped that genealogy would somehow prove he was related to Robert Burns, his favorite poet. He longed to paint the kind of images with his pen that Jill had captured with her brush. He had been writing a few poems along the way to express his deepest thoughts. The most meaningful to print here would be:

The Word Artist

Words are my oils,
The pen my brush.
Prose, pictures I paint.

I'm an outdoor artist.
I sit at my make believe easel
To mind's eye, the view.

Incubated in sleep,
Awakened with desire,
The pen moves effortlessly.

Paper my canvas,
Binding the frame,
An artist nonetheless.

"I was a doctor and healed the sick. Now I'll be a writer and heal the soul. I'll start a book tomorrow to celebrate my 80th birthday. I've already thought of the title….I'll call it *A Trail of Envy*."

Chapter XXXIII

Her Soul Departed

"Future life imagined is seldom future life lived."

The ending of Malcolm's life had to be rewritten. To underline the above profound statement, it was decided to write about what actually took place during the three years spent editing this book.

It would be appropriate for the doctor in light of his long life of trials and tribulations to have another test, perhaps the greatest test of all, of his nobility and ability.

Just as he wrote the final line in his novel, a line he was extremely proud of, a dramatic change was about to occur. He was totally unprepared for this new challenge. He was now 83 years of age and about to celebrate a 37 year anniversary with Jill. When you add the six years that he knew her before marriage you get their 43 year old habit of togetherness. They were an inseparable part of each other, or so he thought. She had been secretly holding back her desire to escape from his disability after that untimely stroke eighteen years earlier. To her, "in sickness and in health" was of no import. Marriage vows be damned. She had found a man who could accompany her on her daily two mile walks. As an added blessing, he was a great dancer. She loved to dance and Malcolm would never be able to accommodate her in that celebratory pastime. This knight on a white charger also was a millionaire. The temptation was too great and as much as she had benefitted from Malcolm's kindness and devotion over all those years, she chose to leave him. The announcement of her intention was sudden, brief, and devastating. Out of the blue, she made her cold, calculated, and heartless speech.

"We have to talk. I want a divorce. My walking partner, Byron, has proposed to me. Why would you want someone who doesn't want you? I want him." With her last remark, she pointed forcefully in the direction of his condominium, as if her mean, spiteful tone of voice was not emphasis enough.

Malcolm was so stunned, he was speechless. He had been sitting on the couch and did not have to pick himself up off of the floor, which would have been impossible in any event, due to his partial paralysis. At least she was kind enough to wait until he was sitting down to attack.

His immediate impulse was to annilate that strange woman sitting across from him. With a verbal sword he wanted to behead her and put her out of her obvious misery. The silence that filled the room was electric and the overwhelming anger rising up from his knotted gut to his brain was thunderous. His ears began to ring. The tinnitus was so loud he put his useful right hand up to cover his ear in an attempt to block it out. He studied her face, which was transfixed in a hateful scowl. Who was this awful woman that had suddenly filled the room with hate? After several moments, he had to admit to himself it was Jill, not the Jill he knew and loved but another Jill that he should have known. The woman that he never dreamed could exist was a selfish, raging, narcisstic, lying bitch. She was heartless.

This affair with Byron had to have been going on for some period of time. Malcolm was clueless. What a lie Jill had been living. A proposal to a married woman was unbelievable deceit. Byron was as heartless as she.

Struck so speechless, Malcolm had the time to see Jill as mindless and pathetic. He was happy she could not read his mind at the moment and subdued his impulsive anger to speak with remarkable clarity and good judgment

"Jill, I am stunned. I love you so much. How could this be? Your agitated state of mind is unreal. Where did that heartless speech come from so spontaneously or was it rehearsed by you and Byron? We need to calm down and talk this situation over for a period of time."

With her arms still flailing the air, Jill's tone continued hysterically. "I'm serious Malcolm. I don't need you anymore. I need him."

"Believe me I know you could not carry on like this unless you are serious. What I am trying to promote here is sanity. It's not so much what you are saying but how you are acting that disturbs me. I got the message. Now give us some time to sort things out and figure how to untangle this mess. We can do this rationally, but it will take time. I am asking you to calm down and give us that time."

Malcolm's rationality at a time like this was surely appropriate but was totally unexpected. Calm medical logic was ingrained in him. Over the next few months he would have to treat Jill as his patient. This would not be too difficult because he had done it so many times in all their years together. The doctor in him would save both of them.

In retrospect, he admitted to himself that Jill had always suffered from low self esteem and he had bolstered her ego so many times. His love for her and his giving nature had made that relatively easy. He promoted and was proud of her beauty and her artistic ability. Relatives from time to time had warned him of her selfish and oft times bizarre behavior. He turned a deaf ear and defended her always. Chronic auto-immune problems had made her his patient as well as his wife. He was her personal day to day physician. Her physical health flourished because of his laser-like medical attention. Her mental state as it turned out was another matter. She later admitted to him during this painful separation period that she had been a victim of incest and had told no one else. Malcolm was unprepared for such an admission but knew instantly that it was the missing piece of the puzzle. She had told him of her experience with rape, but never of her teenaged incestuous experience. He knew she carried that guilt her entire life. Add to that the rape by her first husband on a date that led to pregnancy and a marriage, you get a life of total sexual chaos. Her physical beauty was a curse that led to an ugly mind. Equating rape to a beloved family member and placing the blame on herself totally skewed her mindset. She was a sexual cripple. Malcolm's attempt to fix that with kindness and tenderness was futile, even though he was a masterful and knowledgeable lover. She would compliment him over and over again on his ability to satisfy her sexually. Unknown to him, down deep she was totally unable to appreciate his expertise and his unselfish love. This was tragic, but their relationship did last all those years because of it. She was programmed for short unhappy relationships.

Chapter XXXIIII

The Interim

Malcolm's intuitive knowledge of her plight gave him the unique ability to guide them through this awful time. At first, because of his commitment to love he thought he could change her mind and prevent her from a disastrous remarriage. This greedy other man was a "taker" and not the "giver" she so needed. He feared that her mental state would be made even worse with the added depression and guilt brought on by this pending divorce. Malcolm knew what kind of man would take advantage of such a mentally disabled woman. She was defenseless against Byron's Svengali greed. He had programmed her divorce from Malcolm and would control her new life completely. This would destroy what was left of her low self esteem.

As mentioned above, Malcolm must swallow his pride and use his knowledge of human psychology to attempt the impossible. Lust is hormonal and the strongest of inborn emotions meant to protect the species from extinction. Jill had attracted a lust-filled suitor whose wife had died recently. He was elderly, lonely, and questionably suicidal. This rich man habitually got what he wanted. A retired engineer meant he was pragmatic and goal oriented. Malcolm knew that he would engineer Jill's every move. Moral values and common sense would not prevail here. The good news was that Byron had moved to his winter residence in Arizona and their only connection would be by telephone. He could build his case with astute word directives but at least they would not look into each other's eyes.

Malcolm must woo Jill all over again even though he felt rejected and powerless at this point. Pride would continually rear its ugly head and this battle was all but futile. He had never been a quitter, and he would give it all that he had despite the odds. It certainly didn't help his cause that he was an emotional wreck, teary-eyed, and speechless much of the time.

As part of the separation agreement, Jill promised to come over each morning and stay until six, helping him survive by doing the cleaning, cooking, and laundry. He would greet her with a hug and show his appreciation in every way possible. Much to his surprise, after a couple of weeks she began sitting next to him on the couch and holding his hand.

"I always did admire your hands. They are the hands of a healer," she admitted as they looked into each other's eyes. Whenever he looked into those green eyes, it was instantly and always St. Patrick's Day. The pipes they played, the parade and the happiness marched; the magic of green leprechauns filled his heart. He was buoyant and floated above the ground. His love for her held no boundary, it was pure and deep. St. Patrick's Day had always been near and dear to him because it was his mother and fathers anniversary. Malcolm loved them and they loved him unconditionally.

Holding lips was the natural follow up to this hand holding and closeness. Their kisses were long, deep, and hot. Malcolm's arousal was immediate and obvious. Her smile was mischievous as she extended her hand to help him up from the couch and lead him to the bedroom where they would remain entwined until hunger would drive them to shower and to the living room for dinner. Later she would pace restlessly, give him a good bye kiss, and walk out the door. She would then drive the short distance to Byron's condo to make the daily phone call to Arizona where he waited expectantly at 6:30 pm. Malcolm knew she would paint a much more mundane picture of her daily activities. It would be all cleaning, cooking, and tolerating the disabled old boring husband. Byron would faithfully give her a 6 am wakeup call each morning to fortify her for another day of misery. Again she could expound on her constant mental abuse. Her double life reeked of deceit. Malcolm was convinced her affair with Byron was purely mental to date or he would have been unable to participate in this charade.

The next morning after breakfast, Jill walked slowly toward Malcolm from the kitchen. She was in a trace like state and did not sit down or look at him but stood motionless in front of him. He knew this was an impact moment but had no idea as to why. She continued her vacant stare directed at the rug. Finally she spoke softly in monotone. "I was raped at home when I was thirteen. I have never told this to anyone." Malcolm's well practiced bedside manner kicked in and he spoke with a voice of pure empathy. He had gently grasped her hand that dangled near him. "I am so glad you told me now. You should have shared this with me years ago, I had no idea." He wanted to know more about the circumstances but she didn't offer and he thought it best not to pry. The fact that she was so close with all of her family told him that she blamed herself for this unspeakable wrong she lived with. How very, very sad. There was no time now for him to do anything but feel sorry for her.

At this point, Jill was telling him every detail delightfully about their time apart. It was a bit weird but expected because of her lust driven hormonal state. She was like a teenager again, caught up in an unreal world of fun and expectation of a new life to come with Byron. They planned to do a quick marriage at the courthouse as soon as the divorce was final. Byron had been married only one time for 60 years to his high school sweetheart. Another feather in his cap was his statement to Jill upfront that he thought it immoral to consummate their engagement before that planned quick marriage. To her, he was a man of principle even though he had proposed to a married woman. This strange set of events reassured Malcolm that he had a brief interval to win back his wife and he was making amazing headway in that direction.

To put things in proper perspective and order time wise, we must back up here to those few precious weeks when Jill was coming in daily to help her disabled husband while Byron was far away in Arizona.

Malcolm was still in high hopes that he could get Jill away from her mindset that a divorce and a quick marriage to Byron was inevitable. She seemed to have dramatically softened her stance to the present empathetic mood.

It was shortly before Jill's candid admission of incest that she conceded, "I know Byron and I can't stay here, we will move out right away." She made this concession in all seriousness while holding his hand. Malcolm should have anticipated what the controlling Byron would do, but his emotional state had made him too trusting. He didn't give it a thought that any man would steal his wife and then remain around to be seen with her on a daily basis. He didn't know Byron.

Malcolm's guard was up however, because she had lied to him over and over throughout this sticky prolonged divorce. He concluded immediately that he must have that promise in writing and included in the divorce decree. He was fully aware that the probably fallout of using his immeasurable patience and self control would be getting that decree written in his favor on promises such as this. The chances that he could talk her out of the divorce were remote indeed. He wasn't ready to quit yet however and continued to go along with her unexplainable amorous state of mind.

Their intense lovemaking was enjoyable for him as long as he thought she was changing her mind and that she and Byron had not consummated their love affair. This was physically impossible at present because of Byron's out of state residence and reinforced by his statement earlier that they must wait for marriage. It seemed logical to Malcolm that Byron could salve his conscience with that statement when he had proposed to her even before her divorce was contemplated.

Property settlement and divorce papers had been filed without the use of lawyers at Malcolm's insistence. As a medical doctor, Malcolm knew full well how lawyers prolong and complicate even simple matters. Cost was a factor to be considered as well. Needless to say because of Jill's guilt-ridden conscience, the agreement was very favorable to Malcolm. It was during the three month waiting period that they were enjoying each other's company and he was plotting what other items such as living arrangements would be added at the final court hearing date.

It was now early April and Byron was about to return in one month. Malcolm knew that he had that much time to turn her head. He knew he could no longer heart-wrenching game if Jill was able to meet Byron every night at six o'clock. The fateful letter arrived from the courthouse setting the decree date for June 3rd at 1:30 pm. The parameters were all set, or so he thought until she surprised him with an announcement May 15.

"You're not going to like this, but I have to pick up Byron at the airport this afternoon at 4pm." Her little-girl voice and seeming innocence gagged him.

"Whose idea was it for him to return early?" Malcolm blurted out rudely.

"It was mine." She confessed as she exited the kitchen with his lunch on that damn tray which always reminded him of his disability.

That statement penetrated his chest and stabbed into his heart as if it were a long knife. He knew instantly that this charade must be ended. His impatience with Jill's deceit was long overdue. To explain her shift into so loving a mode as a sign she would stay with him was absurd at this turn of events. It was time to admit that he had been grasping at straws. In bed alone that night he tried to plot out how and when he would dump her.

He did not have domestic help lined up as of yet and was visualizing how frightening it would be ----------------- alone, disabled, and devastated. First he must cement a schedule for a couple of girls he was talking with.

Domestic help would be strange but relatively easy when compared to dealing with a life without Jill at his side and in his bed. At this point the thought was surreal and totally devastating. His panic in regard to such an awful possibility had no doubt been instrumental in forcing him to follow her agenda these past few weeks, but now he must face reality.

His mind was spinning. He could not formulate a complete plan like he normally did and he would play it out day by day. He must sleep and keep a clear head and he willed himself into a restless loss of consciousness.

Byron's arrival on the scene did change things dramatically. Malcolm wanted no part of Jill-Byron and obviously Byron wanted no part of Jill-Malcolm. Jill was now directly in the middle of two suitors. The strain was palpable and her guilt had to be front and center. It was amazing that she continued to placate Malcolm with sexual sweetness.

His mode shifted to devilish psychological warfare now that he had accepted the inevitable. He looked into her eyes while she was trimming his beard and proclaimed triumphantly, "Jill I see it clearly now. He has your heart but I will always have your soul." Malcolm was unprepared for her immediate forthright response. "Darling, you are so right." Shock and surprise quickly turned to melancholy motivating him to write a poem at 4 am the following morning.

The Soul

Protected by the heart
Resting deep inside
The soul that tender part
Where God's hand does reside

Love that lasts through time
Seasons in that far
Fleeting capers seem sublime
Superficial though they are

As the egg of life
Accepting only one
The soul avoids all strife
To hold 'til life is done

A Trail of Envy

My love of four score three
Found a man with temping grace
And did wander off to see
If he could take my place

She knew from the beginning
Her soul was mine to own
They did enjoy a brief inning
To reap tragedy of seeds so sewn.

Chapter XXXV

The Bargain

Dr. McKenna's level-headedness heretofore and throughout the remainder of this painful ordeal would be remarkable for anyone but when you consider he was in his 8th decade of life, it was indeed miraculous.

Another miracle (or was it the work of Malcolm's guardian angel) now presented itself to guide him through this maze. In any event, Jill delivered a message the next morning from Byron. "Byron wants to know how much you would have to spend on help each week to replace me. He wants to help you and get me out of your life quicker. He realizes how hard this must be for you." Jill's delivery of that message was coy and innocent as her proclamations usually were. Byron's deep concern at this point was equally pathetic.

She seemed truly unaware of what a red flag this offer had become for Malcolm. He knew instantly that she was not only speaking for Byron but to their combined effort. It was obvious Byron was being told a tale about her suffering through painful hours helping and enduring Malcolm's rage and helplessness. If Byron had a clue about what was really going on, he would be enraged and seething with anger. Has a knight on a white horse ever been cuckolded? Jill had succeeded in turning everything upside down. Malcolm was being totally informed and her suitor was the victim in this case.

Malcolm was ready to pounce on this opportunity. Now he knew exactly how and when to let go of Jill. He spoke slowly and deliberately. "Jill, tell him I accept this generous offer. If he cuts me a check for $12,000 to be held in escrow by my bank I will release you from your duties after one more week at 6pm Sunday May the 27th. He will be buying four weeks of your commitment if we subtract the two weeks you will be at Elle's to decorate the nursery."

Jill was unprepared for this decisiveness. She looked up in a state of shock. "You can't expect $12,000, are you crazy? That's $3,000 a week!"

"Yes Jill, you have succeeded in making me crazy, but an old money bags has bragged to you about his fortune. Surely $12,000 is pocket change to him. Let's see if he cares about you as much as you think."

Malcolm knew that he was putting Byron in a box. Byron would not dare refuse this offer. Malcolm was laughing inside knowing that he had already planned to let Jill go. Now he was being paid. He had the added satisfaction knowing that Byron was directly prostituting Jill for $3,000 a week. Malcolm took Jill to bed that day for free. After all she was still his wife until June 3rd and not a prostitute to him.

He was confident Jill would be unable to bed Byron until their marriage or at least until after May 27th. That date marked the end of any of his responsibilities for her. His thoughts were turning to how he would lay a guilt trip on Jill by their reliving the past at every opportunity during their final week together.

Chapter XXXVI

The Final Week

As expected Jill returned Monday promptly at eight and elatedly bragged to Malcolm "He's going to cut a check for $12,000."

"I'm shocked!" Malcolm lied, knowing full well what Byron had to do. "We are starting our last week together Jill. Let's make it memorable." He added looking deeply into her eyes. The more memorable he made it, the more he would imprint her guilt for what she had done.

Daily he seized every opportunity to remind Jill of the past and stated over and over "This will be the last time we ever …….." He planned each day's activities to afford these opportunities. On Tuesday he asked her to drive them up the Columbia Gorge, circling back down the Oregon side where they would travel the scenic old highway build in the 1930's by WPA (Roosevelt's Welfare Program). Quaint rock work protected the cars from steep drop offs. Numerous waterfalls spilled down from the high rocky ledges above. The sight was unique and breathtaking. When they first met over 46 years before, he drove her over this awe-inspiring road many times. They would park in solitude, listening to the rushing water and their hearts beating together.

Words of endearment came back to life as they backtracked and reminisced. They parked once again in the exact spot where he had proposed to her 38 years earlier. Tears intermingled as they kissed. His effort to potentiate her guilt took a deep toll on him as well, but he knew he must follow a well conceived plan. All through his life he had done so and even though this torture was perhaps the most painful, he could never relent to be defeated by anyone. Malcolm knew that his future depended on that. In the past it was always his enemies, but this time it was his beloved that wanted to destroy him. The bargain he had made with the devil,

Byron allowed Malcolm to turn rejection around on its rightful owner by rejecting Jill. He must play out this last hand to win an awesome game of survival. He would prove once and for all what a survivor he was.

The next day standing by the couch, beckoning Malcolm to sit there, she spoke unexpectedly and matter of factly "Do you know why I do this? Because I can; and because you are the greatest lover I will ever have. I know how much I will miss that."

He knew that this was one of Jill's rare truthful moments and her impromptu compliment made him happily oblige. He wedged himself in between her soft body and the firm couch arm expectantly. Because the whole day, from the beginning was so emotional, the entanglement of love was appropriately intense.

As they walked down the hall from the bedroom, Jill's dazed expression belied the sincerity of her remark, "Malcolm do you realize that these last several weeks we have made love daily and sometimes even more often? Even young people aren't that crazy. This is unheard of!"

"Oh! I hadn't thought about that Jill. I guess it does prove how deeply I love you. The word 'forever' that you had engraved on my wedding ring meant exactly that to me." Malcolm's quick response capitalized forever.

Forever Love

He had no life, as said she
His mate was dead, hers was me
I had forty years to get it right
He did it zip at a dance one night

I fell for her the day we met
Six years she waited for a marriage set
Two holy men blessed our forever tie
I knew the knot was from the sky

Such history cannot go away
I pray she knows to her dying day
I will take her with me to my death
As I reach for her with my final breath

As they sat together on the couch, for the last time on April the 27th, the finality of it all stabbed her heart with pangs of remorse. She laid her head on his shoulder and he felt tears running down his neck and under his collar. This time it was he who took the initiative and pushed himself up to stand on wobbly legs. When his head cleared enough, he extended his had to her and led her to the bedroom. Emotion was clawing in his skin. Never in his long life had he felt so vulnerable. He was putty in her artist's hands. She molded him into an object of her lust. He was helplessly happy and her fire consumed him. He reveled in her endless orgasm. The moment was so intense that words of pleasure were forced from her enflamed lips in spurts of hot breath. "Oh my God, it is endless, it feeds on itself. Thank you, thank you." They were glued to each other in a never ending embrace and fell into a deep exhausted sleep.

He was awakened with her lips searing his. Slowly those soft coals traveled down to his neck, his chest, and aroused nipples. His back and leg muscles convulsed and he arched to her in ecstasy. She brought him to a second earth shattering climax with her dancing tongue. "Malcolm, you are an ageless wonder. I will never forget you. Please don't forget me."

Their final time together in bed would be unforgettable. It was transcendingly perfect. Unbelievably Shakespeare's "Parting is such sweet sorrow" was played out over and over again on that Sunday when she would leave her car keys and walk away, never to return.

They devoured their last meal together, relieving pains of intense hunger. He had planned it carefully. Her favorite: lobster.

They walked down the hall together at 6 pm, as they had done so many times these past few weeks. This time was punctuated with the finality of an endless deep kiss goodbye. She grasped the doorknob to steady herself as she turned to leave. "Oh, I almost forgot, here." She handed him the ring of keys which included entry to every access door, but foremost, that palm-sized black Lexus key with its gold logo: a logo that she had proudly carried on her water cup, umbrella, and her heart. She loved that car. It was feminine and richly appointed. She had always surrounded herself with such appropriateness. Her tall slender frame was always well draped with clothes carefully chosen and coordinated. Their furniture was equally well chosen and pleasing to her eyes. Malcolm warmly supported her need for such a comfort zone. He was proud of her and somewhat flattered that she included him in her artistic, graceful, and beautiful world. To walk away from all of this made a profound statement within itself.

Walk away she did. He watched from the balcony above as she exited the atrium door, and followed the sidewalk through the quaking aspen trees westward towards Byron's condominium. He knew her eyes were tear-filled as were his. That wetness surrounded him when he called down to her. "Good luck, Jill, and don't forget."

"Forget what?" she answered looking over her shoulder up to where he stood.

"Me." Was his simple heart-rending reply. He watched her look back in his direction repeatedly, until disappearing out of sight never to return again.

Among Our Souvenirs

A final week of love and tears
Made powerful by remorse
Your blindness amid my fears
Impossible your chance of course

I shuffled down the hall
Envying your forceful gait
In the parlor standing tall
Our kiss goodbye my fate

You handed me the keys
To the car and other doors
You, locked out from a life of ease
I, locked in where silence roars

Left intact all our things
For there was no barter
All went the way of the rings
To make yourself a martyr

You have a new lover
His family stuff and cheers
While I hope and recover
Among our souvenirs

Chapter XXXVII

The Decree

The final step in their divorce was to occur in a court appearance on June the 3rd, a date set in stone several weeks before. Jill called at 9 am on that fateful day. This unexpected call was only hours before she had promised to pick him up at 11 am. They were to go to court together as they had done every step of the way to getting their divorce. That call, was like a bomb exploding in Malcolm's ears. She had taken on that mechanical, stern voice once again. "Malcolm, I am not going to pick you up. You really don't need to appear anyway."

"Jill, don't do this now. We have managed to remain friends without lawyers. This is the final step and I do want to be there." He pleaded unabashedly.

"No, I can't come. My advisors have told me so." Jill proclaimed with all the authority she could muster.

Malcolm thought the term 'advisor' was strange. What on earth did that mean? Apparently more than one person and perhaps Byron's lawyer was attempting to sabotage his efforts. He begged her to reconsider, but to no avail. She hung up abruptly.

Fortunately Malcolm had a backup plan in place. He knew that Jill was unstable and that Byron was now calling the shots. He was actually surprised that he had been able to hold Jill's hand and guide her through this divorce settlement thus far. Because of his fear that a blowup could occur at anytime, he had carefully written, dated, and signed the changes that he wanted to present to the judge. This naturally included a specific paragraph concerning Jill's moving out of his neighborhood as well as some financial matters. Malcolm had discussed with his close friend Mary that he would need her help on this day in court. Mary was as compassionate as she was eye catching. She was flawlessly beautiful from head to toe. She had been a lifeline for him throughout this ordeal. Mary was unreal to Malcolm and loveable as any guardian angel could be.

When Jill hung up the phone, he called immediately. "Mary, I'm in trouble. Jill has cancelled out on our trip to court today. Can you come by and pick me up at about 12:30? The court appearance is scheduled at 1:30 pm."

"Of course I will be there Malcolm. This has to be a horrific day for you. Why don't I take you out to dinner afterward?" Mary's voice was soft and supportive in contrast to Jill's put down. It was heaven-sent.

The court appearance was as heartrending as it was momentous. The large room was full of people, all much younger. Malcolm felt very old, resting his chin on his cane, with Mary considerately sitting between he and Jill in the rear corner. He thought this world had gone berserk and everyone was getting divorced. He glanced across at Jill's face starting straight ahead and was somewhat surprised to see large, heavy tears running down her expressionless face. He felt somewhat guilty that his eyes were just as dry as his mouth and throat. He tried to swallow cotton that would not budge. He could not rise when the woman judge entered. A ray of hope crossed his mind, thinking that women judges should be more understanding. She would perhaps be on his side when she learned that Jill was leaving him for another man. The women that had come to his aide, including Mary, felt that any woman who could desert a very old disabled husband was heartless. They were all surprised, chagrined, and guilty by association as members of the female sex.

Malcolm's fears of a long wait on such a hard bench were dispelled when their case was called out first in line. Maybe they took into account his age and those 43 years of marriage. He surmised that all the others in the room must have been teenage marriages breaking up after 8 to 10 years and creating another batch of single moms to fend for themselves. Mary helped him rise and hobble to the table in front of the judge. She remained standing at his left, while Jill seated herself to his right. Mary carried his paperwork up to the bench. Jill had signed it all without question because she was in such a state of surprise that he had arrived early with Mary at his side. Her hopes that he would not appear as her advisors had predicted, were dashed leaving her completely off balance and ashamed.

To Mary's surprise, she had to make several trips back and forth, getting the paperwork in proper legal order. The judge read and asked questions all the while. Finally she said, "You are now divorced."

On hearing that dramatic proclamation, Malcolm's dry eyes gushed forth copious tears. He collapsed onto the table. He felt Jill's hand on his right shoulder and then Mary's on his left, trying to comfort him. They helped him rise and half carried him out of the room where the judge and all those others stared in stunned silence.

Mary was quick to speak with a reassuring statement. "That judge was so compassionate and helpful to your cause. I have never seen or heard of anything like that. Usually you would have had to return with proper paperwork in order." Malcolm, regaining his composure spoke softly, "She was a woman trying to correct the wrongs of this crazy world. Can you believe I still trust women to do that?" He looked directly into Jill's face, where tears were once again flowing. His composure was fortified by having been right about the woman judge.

Mary held Malcolm's arm tightly and helped him walk away from Jill who was the one weak in the knees now. "We'll meet you at the bank to sign the release papers for my check." His confident manner was meant to hit her again while she was on the ropes. He had never been one to return to his corner dejected. He knew the next round always depended on that.

Malcolm was proud to have a beautiful young lady like Mary on his arm for dinner that evening. He smiled to himself thinking how he was a free man only for a few hours and out on a date. Maybe bachelor life would not be so bad after all. He knew this was wishful thinking but enjoyed that fleeting smile nonetheless.

Chapter XXXVIII

In Plain Sight

'Never to return again' sounds sad enough and final enough but as things progressed it became neither sad enough nor final enough.

They had agreed that for Jill and Byron to live in his condo so close to Malcolm would be inhumane. Weeks ago holding hands and looking into each others eyes, Jill conceded "I know we can't stay here, we will move out right away." Malcolm should have anticipated what the controlling Byron would do; but his emotional state made him too trusting. He didn't even consider that any man would steal his wife and then remain around to taunt him. He didn't know Byron.

My View

I look out my windows
The river pleases me
Our circle of buildings
To my right I do see

My eyes pulled to one place
Where my wife and he hides
Behind those walls to cavort
Such horror there resides

A few weeks ago it was
She confessed the affair
She then shared my viewpoint
But now lives where I stare

This view brings reality
Her switch will not die
Devastation my mood
As I stand there and cry

As if to justify and declare to the close knit cove community the magnificence of what he had done, Byron chose to stay with a controversially new bride in his condominium. Sporting their togetherness in plain view somehow made him powerful and helped to subdue whatever conscience he might have in his twisted mind. Malcolm could not bring himself to believe that Jill had any control in her new relationship.

Each day Malcolm's depression and his hatred for Byron deepened. The brazen mockery of it all pounded on him and the thunderous impact was becoming unbearable. To lose Jill, his constant companion of so many years, and to see her so available to another man was tearing him apart.

In World War II, Malcolm had been a rifleman in the infantry. As an avid deer hunter in subsequent years, he maintained his expert marksman status. The thought of a well placed bullet between Byron's eyes, which were now feasting greedily on Jill, haunted him in his sleepless nights. With a scoped 30/30 braced against the railing of his deck, he practiced that shot repeatedly in his mind's eye. Their deck was about 400 yards away with no obstruction between. The condo buildings were placed on a circular drive, giving the deck's such access and made Malcolm's view so heart-rending. Every move they made was clearly visible to him, even from his couch inside.

Jill had become a sun worshipper as was Byron's habit and wore a swimsuit with a short cover up to show off and tan her long shapely legs. He knew her new lover was encouraging this behavior because she had always avoided the sun to protect the delicate skin of her face. A chemical peel, which Malcolm had performed in the past, made her face wrinkle free and vulnerable. Malcolm turned to prolific writing on his novel to keep his sanity through all this torture. His emotional poetry tells a story.

The Wall

In your mind I do not exist
A wall you built to keep me out
Bricks of resentment from the mist
A nefarious excuse of your no doubt

To cover for your newfound lover
A man you barely know
That leap of faith time will uncover
Bitter flaws will surely show

Your bed is made for restless sleep
Enjoy your unknown coming life
Our love climbed hills so steep
Will you survive such future strife?

Life from Ashes

I must admit at long last
That you have left me for another
These great memories of your past
A heavy blanket over me does smother

Do I stand alone to grieve
Does conscious make you share
Where is the door to my reprieve
When each I open sees you there

The loss now appears all mine
Your glory is newfound love
On you the sun does shine
Waiting a verdict from above

Your shady time will surely come
When fate catches up to you
Noble will be my total and sum
A better life will build anew

    His walks, always with his cane, were limited to early mornings when he had the most energy. Byron and Jill apparently slept in so he did not run into them, fortunately. He did, however, meet a woman who recognized him as Jill's ex-husband. She introduced herself and obviously needed to talk. "I'm Sally Benning. I was Byron's girlfriend last year. He wasn't my type for sure and I dumped him. I could tell a lot about your wife and him, but I won't. I just can't imagine what she sees in him. He's a drinker and creates scenes like you wouldn't believe when he is drunk. For a man who professes to have money, he is such a tightwad. He is a terrific dancer though; we went every week to the Elks club. I still go there and see them together. I better shut up now that I have got that off my chest. How are you doing? Everyone around here is so inspired by your spirit and endurance."

Malcolm was fascinated to hear from someone who knew Byron so well and his curiosity made him ask…. "Have you talked to Byron lately?"

"I talked to him at the dance last night. Would you believe, he has the gall to be bragging about how you made the mistake of not putting an exact time frame on their move out? He boasted that he was going to stay as long as he wanted. He said the mountain view from his condo is better than anything on the river. I told him that he had better cool it. I said that you had every right to be thinking about shooting him. He laughed.

Malcolm said she should call him and that they should get together for coffee sometime, all the while expecting that that would not happen. He didn't confess to her that he had considered her outlandish statement about a shooting. He felt less guilt, that she, a bystander, had had the same thought.

Walking the inside loop, away from the river, he did run into Jill as she stopped at the exit gate one morning. Fortunately she was driving alone. She rolled down the window and extended her hand to hold his as she spoke. "I see you walking every morning. You are looking great. How do you feel?" She seemed truly excited to talk. He couldn't help but notice how tan she was in contrast to the white dress she was wearing. Then he turned his gaze and looked into her eyes. "You look great too. I am feeling much stronger these days." Wanting to add "No thanks to you" but thought friendliness would in the long run do more damage.

"By the way, I have a large box of mail for you. Call me when you want to pick it up." He waved goodbye and watched as she drove out of the gate. He was choking back a strong desire to break down and cry. He knew if he did, he would have to sit down and there was no place for that in the middle of the road. He mustered up the strength and courage to hobble back to his building. That evening Jill called. "Byron and I will be over in twenty minutes to get my mail."

"I'm sorry Jill, but you will have to come alone. I don't want him anywhere near me." His voice was emphatic. Oblivious to his feelings, Jill blurted out impatiently, "Forget it then. Goodbye."

Malcolm was puzzling that day, staring out his large picture windows, watching the river when he noticed movement on Byron's deck. Jill had seated herself across the table from Byron instead of on the lounge chair beside him, as was the custom. Byron was waving his arms wildly and doing all the talking. Was this the newlywed's first argument? Their body language was unmistakable.

That silent movie across the way led Malcolm to surmise the soundtrack. Jill had showered Byron with details about meeting Malcolm that morning. She may have mistakenly bragged about his sadness and about how much she knew he still cared for her. Byron smoldered but said nothing. Then when she told him what was said on that telephone call about the mail pick up, Byron blew and instead of going to their usual Wednesday night dance, he confronted her out on the deck. "Get that damned ex-husband out of your head once and for all. I never want to hear his name again." Were the words Malcolm put in the dramatic scene he was watching. A smile of satisfaction buoyed his walk down the hall to his bedroom where he watched TV to forget this day's nightmare.

An hour later, real talking movie on Channel 71, was interrupted by a phone call. Jill's voice was stern, business-like, and demanding. "Don't talk, just listen carefully to me. I don't ever want to talk to or see you again. I hate you. I wish you were dead." The loud thud of a hang up punctuated Jill's obviously rehearsed speech. It was reminiscent of her attack when she had told him of her immediate need for a divorce. Malcolm instantly knew he was right about the deck scene. His mood shifted to total elation and he began to laugh out loud. A real belly laugh. He laughed until he cried, but this time they were tears of joy. Her speech was exactly what he needed to hear. "I'm free at last. I have won this war." He reveled in the thought that Byron was sitting there absorbing every word of that telephone call.

Jill and Byron did move away a short time later. Jill was out of Malcolm's life and he would never speak to her again.

Epilogue

Byron's plan to remain in the cove and taunt Malcolm had boomeranged. He was the victim of his own deceit. Shortly thereafter, the newlyweds moved and Malcolm's victory was complete; if one discounts the loss of his wife. The fact that he had, along the way decided that she must go, makes up for that loss.

Jill had been out of his sight a mere three months and he was already beginning the healing process. He was aided in this regard by a myriad of his close neighbors who were motivated by the cruel audacity of Byron and Jill.

During the next year, Malcolm came to grips with his depression and loneliness. Gradually he realized that he was becoming more independent than he and others dreamed possible. His disability dictated that he have help part time with household upkeep. A small group of dedicated women rallied to that cause. Every one of them grew to respect and love Malcolm and his plight.

The greatest healer in all of this was his innate ability to write poetry and novels. He always had one girl and her laptop to potentiate this passion. Several novels, including his autobiography and a book of poems were the byproduct of his need to have a life. His plan was to produce the product and not get bogged down with attempts at publication, which he deemed burdensome and awesomely impossible. His success in life had always depended on an ability to compartmentalize. He would divide and conquer; take it one day at a time, restoring his battered ego. He debated with himself as to whether the final chapter in his life would include a small group of paid care-giving women who he would love as his family along with his six children or an unlikely alternative.

The alternative of course, would be one woman to love and cherish. He was capable of, and in his heart wanted that woman, but did such a unique woman exist? She would have to be introspective and sensual enough to appreciate this guru-like, intense, loving man. His never ending flame could incinerate most feminine, fragile moths.

The odd-shaped piece in the puzzle that was missing not only existed but had been known to him for well over a year. Elizabeth Roth was a real estate agent with whom he had spoken to on his visit with his son in Arizona during that first Christmas away from Jill. The fortuitous phone call lasted about an hour because she was friendly and so easy to talk to. He told her of his plight and he understood that she had a horse but no man. He had no email access but received a hand written note with a business card enclosed shortly after he returned home. Her handwriting was as warm as her voice. Malcolm who was an expert graphologist appreciated that. She was expecting that he might buy a condo in Cave Creek near his son's home, but his thoughts were about an attractive pen pal. Within a week he had composed a well thought out letter. In that masterpiece, he told her all about herself and how in the past he had hired office help based not only on interview, but on their handwritten letters. He flattered her by telling her that on that basis, he would have hired her. He even included a recent poem to emphasize that he was a writer of sorts. He was very disappointed when no answer to his long belabored letter appeared in his mail over the next few weeks. He said aloud to himself one afternoon while walking back upstairs from the mailbox, "I guess I am not the writer I thought I was or maybe she was offended by my audacity. I assumed we were old friends even though we had never met. Oh well. I sure tried."

He was vindicated a couple of weeks later when a red envelope with distinctive handwriting appeared. "Why now?" He asked himself. Her letter was not long, but it was not businesslike either. She thanked him for his letter and especially liked the handwriting analysis and the poem, but it was the last line that caught his eye and he dwelled on it for several days. It popped into his head over and over again. "Anyway, just a note to say 'hi'! Warm regards, Beth."

It was unique and friendly to end a letter with "hi". His writers mind read a bundle into that simple word and he told her as much in his reply. This time around he did not anticipate a quick response but he knew she would when her wild spirit moved her. He liked her nonchalance and his persistence could win in the end.

Gradually during the coming year their correspondence reached Elizabeth Barrett Browning proportions. She was intrigued, not by his penmanship, but by his carefully chosen words. They were destined to meet. Was it an omen that both women were named Elizabeth?

He met her for the first time when she arrived on flight 1427 at the Portland Airport on a magnificent summer day. She was older than her business card photograph but even more beautiful. Her tall slender frame and healthful Arizona suntan gave her well chosen white business suit catalog style. Handwriting had understated her presence. She was breathtaking.

Malcolm was suddenly struck inadequate. For him, his age and disability cast a dark shadow over this long anticipated meeting. She quickly dispelled these fears when she hurried directly toward him. Her open arms encircled him as she planted a light warm kiss on his lips. "You are exactly as I had imagined. The white hair and beard makes you look the part of the silver fox that I know you to be. You read my handwriting but I read your brain writing. You are a renaissance man. Your combined medical and literary intellect is overwhelming. You intimidate with such a flawless memory and common-sense grasp of life." The tone of her voice was genuine and no way solicitous giving Malcolm a surge of courage and renewed strength.

They walked to the baggage area arm in arm and their conversation from then on was nonstop fun. The feelings he had for her from a distance were reinforced and more intimate now that they were close. He was in love but dare he think this gorgeous, classy lady felt the same? An aura of youthful charm surrounded this mature beauty and the sight of her would bedevil any man. He showed her the guest bedroom in his magnificent condo, with the breathtaking view of the Columbia River. She was impressed and told him so in glowing terms. This was her style; you always knew where she was coming from. He appreciated such honesty, which mirrored his own.

She helped him put together lunch but couldn't wait to delve into his writings. Starting with the leather bound volume where he had written most of his poems, she was entranced. Written words were everywhere; scattered on various legal pads and ring bound notebooks.

"I had no idea you had written so much. Oh, I really like this one called April Fool. I like all of your poetry, it is so thought provoking." Her enthusiasm lifted his spirits. He could not take his eyes off of her while she was so distracted. Beth was an intriguing package of beauty and brains.

"I'll show you the three novels later." He offered with a twinkle in his eye knowing how impressed she would be with the sheer volume of his efforts.

"Malcolm, we will have to work on publishing all this. I have many high up contacts in my native New York City. I recall you wrote me that you haven't made efforts in that direction to date."

"That's right Beth, I haven't. I knew you escaped New York to take refuge in Arizona but I really don't know much about those years back east. We have so much to talk about." Malcolm's excitement at their being together at last was telegraphed in the tone and eagerness of his voice. Beth was likewise overwhelmed and their excitement kept them awake until after two a.m. They were both highly motivated for a prolonged embrace in the hallway. Their eyes locked in deep searching, promised a magical goodnight kiss. Her lips melted, filling his body with a warm glow of complete surrender. Their eyes held as she turned to the right to her bedroom and he turned to the left to his. The kiss, lingering in his mind, reassured him that she was as serious about their relationship as he was. He fell into bed exhausted, exhilarated, and totally happy. He was whole again.

Beyond his wildest dreams, Beth complimented and completed his life. She had been a very big wheel in the New York City machinery, and promoted her man as no one else could. He had judged her letter writing correctly, she was very capable of helping him edit and rewrite his novels. They became a team and created books together. Her feminine viewpoint greatly enhanced the romantic scenes and their own romance added an intense emotional touch. Inseparable, like the pages of the stories they wrote, happiness surrounded and nurtured their relationship. He became a world famous, published writer. One of life's many circles closed finally after 63 years. McKenna vividly thought back to Germany, when he was 19 and walking along some road in a very long line of troops, as the infantry always did. An artillery unit was travelling through when a voice from one truck shouted repeatedly.

"McKenna, who is McKenna?"

When Malcolm turned and walked toward the truck, an officer hopped down and greeted him excitedly.

"I found your diary a few weeks ago and have been looking for you every since. Here it is. I know how important it must be to you. You are quite a writer. When this war is over, that's what you should do---------write."

That moment had been magic and unforgettable. It was as though the constant grinding painful motion of war stopped. With Beth's' help, McKenna had at last become that writer. Beth was that 'giver' he had never before experienced and their 'giver-giver' relationship lasted for the rest of his very long life.

Malcolm's plans promoting Jill to become a world famous artist were interrupted when she chose to divorce him. It is ironic, that because of her betrayal, he became a world famous author and was finally back on his life-long trail of envy. Those who believe in karma smile and gleefully say:

"We told you so."